The Healing Plants
of the Celtic Druids

The Ancient Celts and their Druid healers
used plant medicine to treat the mind, body
and soul

The Healing Plants of the Celtic Druids

The Ancient Celts and their Druid healers used plant medicine to treat the mind, body and soul

Angela Paine

MOON
BOOKS

Winchester, UK
Washington, USA

First published by Moon Books, 2018
Moon Books is an imprint of John Hunt Publishing Ltd., No. 3 East Street, Alresford
Hampshire SO24 9EE, UK
office1@jhpbooks.net
www.johnhuntpublishing.com
www.moon-books.net

For distributor details and how to order please visit the 'Ordering' section on our website.

ISBN: 978 1 78535 554 7
978 1 78535 555 4 (ebook)
Library of Congress Control Number: 2017947361

A CIP catalogue record for this book is available from the British Library.

Design: Stuart Davies

Printed and bound by CPI Group (UK) Ltd, Croydon, CR0 4YY, UK

We operate a distinctive and ethical publishing philosophy in
all areas of our business, from our global network of authors to
production and worldwide distribution.

Contents

Also by Angela Paine: The Healing Power of Celtic Plants

Acknowledgements

First and foremost I owe a huge debt to John Daniell, who spent hours scanning in and cleaning up the botanical drawings of the plants in this book, who provided me with books on archaeobotany, pollen core analysis, the history of the vegetation of Britain in the time of the ancient Celts and many more. He read the final version of the book, making many useful suggestions. My heartfelt thanks go to Nimue Brown, who encouraged me to write a second book of Celtic healing herbs and answered all my stupid questions over the past year, patiently and speedily; and also to Trevor Greenfield and the rest of the team at Moon Books. Helena Petre helped me overcome the initial inertia that was preventing me from approaching my publisher, John Hunt. I am grateful, as always, to the lovely librarians at Stroud Library, for acquiring rare and expensive books for me to borrow and to my niece, Clara, for acquiring many of the scientific papers that I referred to in the book.

Part I: Introduction

Chapter 1

Why I Wrote this Book

In 1991 I went to the Palazzo Grassi in Venice, to see an exhibition: The Celts, under the scientific direction of Sabatino Moscati. This was a quarter of a century ago but the memory lingers on of a wonderful display of Celtic artefacts from twenty-four countries, covering a period of one thousand years from 600 BCE. The exhibition was an Aladdin's cave of enormous golden torques, bracelets and earrings, bronze and terracotta vessels, bowls and cups, bronze and iron belts and helmets, iron swords and shields, chariots and statues, of exquisite craftsmanship, all decorated with swirling, elegant Celtic designs. Leafy tracery and stylised animals spoke volumes about the interconnectedness of life, both plant and animal. These objects made up a poetic ode to nature, honouring all living things, including forests, tribal goddesses and powerful beasts. I was transported to an ancient time when the world was full of trees and animals, all sacred and important in their own right when humans did not value themselves more highly than their environment. Though they left almost nothing written down, the ancient Celts expressed their beliefs through designs which capture the essence of the horse, the tree, the deer, the wild boar, the ram, the stork, the eagle, the bull, rather than trying to depict an exact replica, as the Romans did. There were many mythological animals, such as horned serpents with fish tails, as well as dragons and abstract designs and even a little golden votive boat from Ireland. The exhibition traced the sphere of influence of the ancient Celts from 600 BCE onwards, their culture, language and way of life, right across Europe. There were representations of mistletoe, madder, woad and yew, all plants with spiritual significance. The sheer quantity of beautiful objects on display made a lasting impression on me and left me feeling that the Celts were a highly cultured people, intimately connected with their environment.

At the time I was carrying out my PhD research into the tropical plants used to treat tropical diseases at the London School of Pharmacy. On obtaining my doctorate I left London and academia and went to live on the borders of Wales. I studied and grew the native healing herbs, eventually teaching a small group of students and travelling round the country giving talks about the subject. Repeated requests for a book on Celtic herbs led to my writing *The Healing Power of Celtic Plants*. I chose from an array of plants mentioned in the Physicians of Myddvai's thirteenth-century Welsh herbal, the earliest British secular herbal that I could find. From this selection I focussed on those that were growing in Britain at the time of the ancient Celts, during the first millennium BCE, as evidenced by samples of pollen from that era. Then from this collection I selected a few that herbalists, and in some cases doctors, still use today. I looked at the research that had been carried out on these plants, investigated their chemical constituents and noted how these affect the human body. I analysed the results of clinical trials that looked at the effect some of these plants had on groups of patients and demonstrated that if herbal medicine is used correctly it can be effective in curing a number of conditions.

Years have passed since my first book was published and there has been a great deal of new archaeological research as well as research in the field of medicinal plant chemistry. I began to think that it was time to explore some more of the plants that may have been used as medicine by the ancient Celts.

Exciting New Discoveries about the Ancient Celts of Britain

When I was researching *The Healing Power of Celtic Plants*, people generally believed that the Celts originated in central Europe and migrated west, south west and north from there. But J. T.

Koch's research published in 2013 and 2014 revealed that Celtic languages evolved much earlier, all along the westernmost edge of Europe. Archaeologists found inscriptions dating back to 700 or 600 BCE on tombstones. These inscriptions were carved in an ancient Phoenician writing system. These languages from the Bronze Age in northern Spain matched the languages spoken in Brittany, Cornwall, Wales, Ireland and Scotland. This suggests that the people who we now call Celts evolved gradually along the far west coasts of Europe, over a much longer period than we previously thought. It seems that they did not come from Germany and invade Britain. They were already in Britain, building their hill forts, trackways, hut settlements, stone circles and standing stones. Caesar, one of the first people to refer to 'The Celts' was probably referring to Brittany when he wrote that only one part of Gaul was Celtic and the people who lived there called themselves Celts. The many different tribes who lived in Britain at that time did not call themselves Celts, rather referring to themselves as Iceni, Atrebates, etc., but they all spoke Celtic languages, languages which are still spoken today by two million people in Wales, Ireland, Scotland, Cornwall and Brittany. It was not until 1703 that Paul-Yves Pezron coined the term Celtic to describe this group of languages and the people who spoke them.

Britain was as densely populated in the Iron Age as it was at the time of the Doomsday Book, according to field archaeologist David Miles. We can see evidence of this in the more sparsely occupied areas of Britain, such as Wales, where traces of ancient settlements have survived the ravages of urban sprawl. Almost six hundred Iron Age hill forts, the largest covering an area of over six hectares, are strung out along the Welsh Marches from Moel Hiraddug in the North to the Severn Estuary in the South. The ancient Celtic tribes who built these hill forts formed a rich, powerful and highly organised civilisation, as described by Andouze and Buchsenschutz in their book, *Towns, Villages and*

Countryside of Celtic Europe.

Farming, Mining and Trade in Ancient Celtic Britain

David Miles discovered that tribes living in the area around the white horse of Uffington had carved it into the hillside in 800 BCE. This wonderful spiritual design elevated the horse to a sacred being, high up on the hillside. He found that the land below this talisman was divided into large parallel blocks or parishes, each giving the people access to river, meadow, arable land, woodland and pasture. This gave him an insight into the way the ancient Celts farmed the land. They were so successful at growing wheat, barley and spelt, which they stored in large underground silos, capped with clay, that they exported it to Gaul (modern day France). We can still see the remnants of their settlements, boundaries and trackways in aerial photographs. They mined the rich deposits of copper and tin in Cornwall and Devon, which their imaginative and creative metal smiths fashioned into some of the lovely objects that I saw in the Palazzo Grassi in Venice.

In 2002 Barry Cunliffe, drawing on the writings of Diodorus, wrote an account of the journey of Pythias the Greek in 300 BCE. Diodorus said in his Library of History:

> The inhabitants of Britain who live on the promontory called Belerion are especially friendly to strangers and have adopted a civilised way of life because of their interaction with traders and other people. It is they who work the tin ... and convey it to an island which lies off Britain called Ictis, for at the ebb tide the space between this island and the mainland becomes dry and they can take the tin in large quantities over to the island on their wagons. (And a peculiar thing happens in the case of the neighbouring islands which lie between Europe and Britain, for at flood-tide the passage between them and the mainland runs full and they have the appearance of

islands, but at ebb tide the sea recedes and leaves dry a large space and at that time they look like peninsulas.) On the island of Ictis the merchants buy the tin from the natives and carry it from there across the Strait of Galatia (the Channel) and finally, making their way on foot through Gaul for some thirty days, they bring the goods on horseback to the mouth of the Rhone.

Pythias the Greek travelled all the way to Britain in 300 BCE, through France along the Rhone, then probably on foot or on horseback as far as the English Channel, which he crossed in a small boat. He travelled along the south coast of Britain in a series of little boats, stopping frequently to leave the coast and walk inland where he described the people he met. He continued his journey along the west coast of Wales and all the way up to the coast of Scotland. His writings have been lost but various contemporaries read them, including Diodorus, from whom we have this information about the ancient Celts who lived along the Southern coast of Britain. The promontory of Belerion was the Penwith peninsula of Land's End. The island of Ictis may have been St Michael's Mount, since it is near to the tin mines of Cornwall and cut off at high tide. Or it could have been Mount Batten in Plymouth Sound because archaeologists found a lot of late Bronze Age metalwork and Iron Age objects here. Mount Batten was a major trading port at the time of Pythias.

David Miles's research revealed that the ancient Celts living along the south coast of Britain traded indirectly with Rome. Most of the trade went on between the tribes in Britain, who exported iron, tin and copper, and the tribes in Gaul, from whom they imported wine, figs, olive oil and glass. Strabo added that the Celts also traded hides, corn, hunting dogs and slaves. The Celts in Britain used little wicker boats covered in hide, rather like the curraghs that are still in use off the coast of Galway, which are now covered in tarred canvas, and just like the little golden votive boat that I saw in the exhibition in Venice. These boats had both oarsmen and a sail, and they seem to have used them to transport goods along the coast of Britain, though they may also have crossed the Channel. Pythias probably travelled in these little boats, which must have been quite frightening once he got up to the wild and windy coast of Scotland. The Celtic tribes in Gaul had slightly larger boats so they may have been the ones who crossed the Channel to trade with the Celtic tribes in Britain. They continued trading across Gaul, using the rivers part of the way, until they reached the Mediterranean and from here they traded with Rome. And so it was that the ancient Celts of Britain who lived along the south coast had access to Mediterranean goods, ideas and plants, both edible and medicinal.

Places of Worship of the Ancient Celts

The ancient Celts used rivers as routes across the country to avoid the impenetrable forest that covered most of the land. They and their Druids revered rivers, springs and wells, which were associated with healing and fertility, according to Anne Ross. The rivers in Britain were named after goddesses: Dee (Deva), Clyde (Clota), Severn (Sabrina), Braint of Anglesea and Brent of Middlesex (Brigantia). Aqua Sulis at Bath was named after the life-giving mother Celtic Goddess Sulis. (The Romans, who recorded all these names romanised them so we do not have a record of the actual Celtic river Goddesses' names.) The ancient Celts made offerings to these goddesses of all sorts of valuable iron and bronze objects, such as swords, shields, cauldrons, coins, brooches, pottery, shrine bells, throwing them into lakes and rivers, much to the delight of the marauding Romans who stole much of this treasure. But the Celts threw such an enormous quantity of offerings into the water that hoards still come to light from time to time. For example in 1958 Fox described the hoards recovered from the rivers Thames, and Withal in Lincolnshire. The ancient Celts also threw animal and human bones (possibly whole animals and humans) into rivers and lakes.

The ancient Celts dug shaft wells, which they regarded as entrances to the otherworld. Anne Ross describes one of the earliest shaft wells, excavated in 1962, two miles from Stonehenge and cut through the chalk one hundred and ten feet down, terminating in a well with remnants of wooden buckets and ropes and pieces of Bronze Age pottery. Stokes spoke of the otherworldly Conlla's Well in the Prose Tales in the Rennes Dindshenchas. This well had a wise hazel tree growing beside it, who scattered her magic hazel nuts into the water. These fed the sacred salmon who lived in the well and acquired supernatural wisdom by eating the nuts. Convention's well had fourteen thousand coins in it, together with an assortment of bronze and gold objects.

The ancient Celts and their Druids revered all kinds of trees, recognising their importance in making the rain fall. Lucan described the sacred groves where they performed ceremonies and rites, sometimes under a particularly venerable tree. Ancient tree worship has filtered down to the present day through the myths and tales of Wales and Ireland, in which the heroes' and heroines' names incorporate the names of trees. Mac Cuill means son of Hazel, Mac Cuillinn: son of Holly, Mac Ibar: son of Yew, Guidgen: son of wood, Guerngen: son of Alder and Dergen: son of oak. Stokes describes several sacred trees: Tortu's Tree, an ash, Eo Rosa, Eo Mugna, both yews and the ash Tree of Dath. He describes the mythical tree of Mugna, an ancient yew which bore acorns, apples and nuts and whose top was as broad as the plain it stood on. This is similar to the marvellous oak on a plain, described in the Mabinogion, where the Welsh God Lleu took refuge after his death, when he transformed himself into an eagle and flew up into its branches. In 1834 Williamson discovered oak branches in an oak coffin in a tumulus at Gristhorpe near Scarborough which suggested that the oak was one of the most sacred trees of the ancient Celts. Trees were so important that the first people to work metal to form minute detailed reliefs in Britain often surrounded the heads they carved with leaf crowns, or blended the heads into a leafy background, as described by Jacobsthal in 1944.

The forests of Britain teemed with animals, including bears, wolves, otters; and the trees were filled with birds. The ancient Celts held all animals in awe as demonstrated by the stone statues, bronze ornaments, shields, silver and gold jewellery that depict them. The stag was particularly important, hence the horned God, Cernunnos, who may have come from Scandinavia, where he was particularly venerated, but was taken up by the British Celts. The horned god was concerned with fertility, wealth and commercial prosperity. His chthonic symbols, serpent, ram, stag and bull are all associated with wealth. The serpent who emerges from the earth is associated with the otherworld. The ancient Celts knew that wealth was underground. They dug deep mines to find copper, iron and tin, so associated underground with the otherworld, with wealth, danger and death. The Christian church did their best to eradicate Cernunnos, since he was concerned with fecundity both human and animal, hence his transformation into the horned Satan. The church similarly demonised the serpent.

The ancient Celts performed ritual and ceremony at burial sites such as grave mounds. Tara in county Meath in Ireland is one such place, where the tribes gathered together to honour their divine ancestors, according to Anne Ross. Burial mounds provided another entrance to the otherworld and were places of magic, as demonstrated by the Irish Dindshenchas myth: Len Linfiaclach was a craftsman who lived in a lake and made bright vessels for Fland, the daughter of Flidais, the goddess of wild things. Each night, after he had finished work he would throw his anvil east towards the burial mound, scattering a shower of water, fire and purple gems as it flew through the air.

The ancient Celts used ritual sanctuary enclosures, ritual pits and roofed shrines, and according to Anne Ross, archaeologists have found remnants of these in various places in Europe and Ireland. Recently archaeologists have made exciting new discoveries that demonstrate that the whole area around Stonehenge is full of ancient religious structures, far more ancient than the iconic stone circle itself. On the 6th September 2015 David Keys, writing for the *Independent*, described the Stonehenge Hidden Landscapes Project, led by Professor Vince Gaffney of Bradford University and Professor Wolfgang Neubauer of the Ludwig Boltzmann Institute in Vienna. The survey used ground penetrating radar, magnetometry and electro-magnetic induction to investigate five square miles around Stonehenge. They found more than twenty previously unknown ancient shrines and sacred enclosures, including a Stone Age temple, near what is now the village of Durrington, in Wiltshire. This huge horseshoe-shaped temple was built more than one thousand years before Stonehenge and was made up of at least two hundred large standing stones, most of them three metres tall and one and a half metres wide. The temple faced Beacon Hill, a sacred landmark. People the world over who practise the most ancient indigenous religious traditions have sacred sites where they perform ceremonies, which are often hills or mountains, so it is likely that Beacon Hill was one such sacred site.

On November 18th 2016 David Keys, again writing for the *Independent*, described the latest discovery of the Stonehenge Hidden Landscapes Project, a huge, prehistoric religious and ceremonial complex at Larkhill, Wiltshire. It was built in 3650 BCE, one thousand years before Stonehenge and consisted of 950 metres of segmented ditches in two great concentric circles. Clearly this was an ancient temple. So far archaeologists have discovered about seventy of these ancient circular ditch complexes in Britain and there were probably many more. Unfortunately no one can visit this ancient monument because the area is covered by modern military buildings and is fenced off and not open to the public. However, the archaeologists were allowed in to excavate this wonderful structure and they found fragments of smashed bowls and cattle bones in the ditches. The ancient people performed rituals, ate large quantities of beef and deliberately smashed the ceramic bowls. They also found fragments of human skull bones. There were probably more than two hundred bowls and the bones of dozens of slaughtered cattle from a succession of feasts in the complex's ditches. These were sacrificial offerings. The monument appears to have been revered for millennia. A leading Wessex Archaeology prehistorian, Matt Leivers, said: 'The newly found site is one of the most exciting discoveries in the Stonehenge landscape that archaeologists have ever made. It transforms our understanding of the intensity of early Neolithic activity in the area.'

If archaeologists were to survey the rest of Britain using the techniques used by the Stonehenge Hidden Landscapes Project, many more ancient temples and shrines would probably come to light. We already know of an Iron Age Celtic temple at Heathrow, described by Grimes, which the Romans razed to the ground. We also know of an Iron Age temple of the Coritani Celtic tribe, described in the *Times* on October 21, 1963. After the Romans invaded they tended to destroy everything sacred to the Celts, including their temples, and to build Roman temples in their place.

The Role of the Druid in Ancient Celtic Britain

Ronald Hutton said: 'The Druids may well have been the most prominent magico-religious specialists of some of the peoples of north-western Europe just over a couple of thousand years ago.' 'They were,' he continued 'as sophisticated in their organisation as in their knowledge, having different divisions of expertise served by specialists with different names.' Bards, or poets; Ovates, who prophesied; and Druids, who were the priests, shamans, philosophers and judges, according to Greek and Roman writers. 'They had an annual meeting,' Ron Hutton said, 'in which Druids from all the different tribes of a particular region assembled to discuss matters of common interest.' This echoes the annual meetings of the Pueblo people of New Mexico, which still occur today and which representatives of all the remaining tribes in the US attend. According to Julius Caesar the Druids virtually ruled Britain, since they were its lawmakers. Caesar said that Druids were concerned with 'divine worship, the due performance of sacrifices, public and private and the interpretation of ritual questions'. He said that all the Druids recognised the authority of a single leader, who held the post for life. They carefully observed the natural world around them and performed religious ceremonies in the open for everyone to see, only retreating to the forests after the Roman invasion. Many people say that the Welsh poets are the heirs of the bards, preserving their traditions, which would account for the relatively high status of present-day poets in Wales.

Although many believe that the Druids wore long, white robes, as described by Pliny, Sjoestedt describes the chief Druid of Ireland wearing a bull's hide and a white speckled bird's headdress with fluttering wings, a very shamanic description more in keeping with the shamanic role of the Druid. They communed with the spirit world, or "otherworld", gaining prophetic insights and valuable knowledge about the illness they had been asked to heal, according to John and Caitlin Matthews, just as the shamans of native peoples throughout the world still do today. The ancient Celts believed that all aspects of the natural environment were possessed of spirit, including rocks, water, trees, animals, birds and fishes, and all belonged to the otherworld. Iron Age Britain and probably Stone Age Britain were numinous worlds, where everything was imbued with spirit, according to Aldhouse-Green. Every aspect of the natural world was precious to the ancient Celts and their Druids, especially trees and many of the forest trees were enchanted: the Willow, with her water-trailing branches and healing bark, the Yew with his seductive, dark, death-like enchantment, the Elder with her sweet blossoms filling the air with heady perfume, to lure men to the world of fairy, from thence never to return. It was a world where spirit was ever present, and nothing was quite as it seemed.

Caesar said, 'It is said that the doctrine of the Druids was invented in Britain and was brought from there into Gaul; even today those who want to study the doctrine in greater detail usually go to Britain to learn there.' This ties in with the current view that the Celtic languages and culture evolved along the western coasts of Europe, including Britain. He said: 'They do not think it right to commit their teachings to writing.' Originally for two reasons: they did not want their doctrines to fall into the wrong hands and they did not want their pupils to rely on the written word and so neglect to train their memories. It does not follow that the ancient Celts did not have a written language. Recent discoveries in Spain and Portugal show that an ancient Celtic language existed, which was used to inscribe tombstones. According to Anne Ross, the ancient Celts expressed themselves obliquely and indirectly. This shows in their art, as well as in the highly idiomatic Celtic languages which are still in use today. Ancient Celtic traditions, faiths and remedies have remained far longer where people continued to express themselves in these languages, which make the traditional literature of Wales and Ireland particularly rich depositories of Celtic belief and customs. The ancient Druids may well have been able to read and write, both in Celtic languages and Latin and Greek; and medical texts from ancient Greece and Rome could well have reached them. Caesar had heard that Druid students or apprentices had to learn long poems by heart and that they studied and trained for twenty years. He also said that Druids had 'many discussions concerning the stars and their movement, the size of the cosmos and the earth, the world of nature, the powers of deities' and taught all this to their students. He said the Celts worshipped a god of healing, a goddess of arts and crafts, a god who ruled over the sky, a war god and a god of arts, travel and commerce, who was the most popular. He said they had magnificent funerals in which they burnt everything belonging to the deceased, along with their corpse.

Caesar also said, 'The Druids attach particular importance to the belief that the soul does not perish but passes after death from one body to another; they think that this belief is the most effective way to encourage bravery because it removes the fear of death.' This sounds a little sceptical but then despite his admiration for their wisdom, Caesar saw the Druids as agitators, stirring up foci of resistance against him in Gaul. Celtic tribes from Britain did cross the Channel to help their fellow Celts fight the Romans. It is likely that they sympathised with their fellow tribesmen who were trying to preserve their culture and religion and didn't want the Romans to impose their spirit-denying, Roman-Emperor-glorifying religion on them. Ronald Hutton said: 'Patriotic Druids were there to inspire their people to resist invaders and preserve their identity as free inhabitants of a land that they had made their own from time immemorial. Spiritually, they were part of an organic relationship with the natural world within which they lived and which would itself be, by implication, polluted and damaged by its conquest at the hands of brutal foreigners.'

Druids and Druidesses were responsible for the well-being, physical, mental and spiritual of the people. Many historians, including Jean Markale, describe women as equal with men in Celtic Britain, where women could and did achieve high status. In 60 CE there were women rulers in Britain, notably Cartimandua, queen of the Brigantes and Boudicca, queen of the Iceni, as well as Druidesses. During the Iron Age important women were buried in rich female tombs, all over Europe. The most impressive is at Vix in Burgundy, where a woman adorned with golden jewellery, including a solid gold torc, was buried beneath a six-metre high, forty-two-metre diameter burial mound, accompanied by a huge bronze wine mixing flagon. Andre Pelletier, in La Femme dans la Société Gallo-Romaine, suggests that the lady from Vix was a priestess or prophetess. E. Champlin talks about a rich chariot burial of a mid Iron Age woman in Yorkshire, who was buried with a mirror, something rare at that time. She may have been a shaman, or Druidess, since people with mirrors were two spirit persons, who could operate in this and the spirit world.

Ancient Celtic Medicine

A study of native peoples the world over reveals that all share a common animistic view of life and their environment and all have priest-like figures: shamans, curanderos or witch doctors, traditional healers who perform ceremonies, heal the sick with plants, prophesy and act as judge in the same way as the Druids did. Both Druids and Druidesses probably studied the healing properties of plants, made healing potions and performed ceremonies, just as the native healer, or curandero, in South America does today, as described by Zethelius and Balick in 1982. Balick, an American ethnobotanist, explains how the spiritual qualities of the plants are as important as their physical properties. Observing native healers the world over, we can deduce that the Druids knew the healing properties of hundreds of plants, observed the effect of each plant on their patients and fine-tuned their medical art over generations. It is likely that they spent long hours meditating and developing their powers of intuition and inspiration. According to Efren C del Pozo: 'Indigenous pharmacology is always based on empiricism; however, magic procedures and religious ceremonies are often mixed in medical use.' To this day shamans throughout the world mix the herbs they give their patients, keeping the active ingredients a secret, only revealing it to their apprentice, and accompanying the medicine with a ceremony. It is likely that the Druids similarly only revealed which plants they used to treat their patients to one carefully chosen apprentice, performing ceremonies as part of the patient's treatment. Long after the Druids ceased to exist, country women continued to use herbs and incantations to treat the sick and it was these women who were accused of witchcraft, burnt at the stake and drowned by the Catholic Church during the Middle Ages. The ancient Celts treated the patient as a whole, but considered that the cause of an illness could be physical, mental or spiritual. Spiritual sickness was the most severe, resulting in soul loss, causing the patient to lose interest in life, even lose consciousness, go into a coma and die. Robert Graves describes how Druids travelled to the otherworld to retrieve lost souls, just as native shamans do in many parts of the world today, as described by Michael Balick.

The Druids brewed their herbal concoctions in giant cauldrons in the forests and wild places. Caitlin and John Matthews say that the cauldron was a symbol of inspiration, knowledge, wisdom and rebirth and its magic powers are described in Celtic myth. Shakespeare's three witches on the moor with their cauldron were the descendants of the Druids, foretelling the future and frightening those who came near.

The Celts believed in working hard and playing hard during their numerous festivals throughout the year. Although drunkenness was condoned during festivals, overeating was seriously frowned on. This is reflected in the Physicians of Myddfai's herbal, whose remedies are punctuated by frequent exhortations to eat sparingly:

Whosoever would prolong life, should restrain his appetite, and not eat over abundantly.

Whosoever, restraining their appetite, refrain from gluttony and eat slowly, these shall live long.

If you eat simple food it will be more easy for the stomach to digest it.

When you eat, do not eat away all your appetite but let some desire for food remain.

Do not eat, til the stomach has become empty.

The Physicians of Myddvai also advised people to drink plenty of spring water for its miraculous health-giving qualities. Sacred springs, which can still be found throughout Britain, often have carved stone basins to collect the water and were kept clean, free of vegetation and animals. The Celts bathed in the sacred springs and rivers, in much the same way as the Hindus bathe in the many sacred rivers in India, including the Ganges. According to David Miles, they built bridges and causeways over rivers for ceremonies, which they performed during lunar eclipses.

Chapter 2

The Plants: How to Recognise, Find, Grow, Preserve and Use Them

Recognising the Herbs

In the time of the ancient Celts, when people lived in close contact with nature, children were taught to recognise the plants which surrounded their homes from an early age. However, with the age of industrialisation, whole swathes of the population, forced to leave their land by the enclosure acts, to work in the new mills and factories, gradually lost this knowledge. Plant recognition became the field of expert botanists, who developed a huge terminology to describe the minute differences between different plants. They divided plants up into kingdoms, divisions, subdivisions, classes, orders, families, tribes, genera and species in a somewhat militaristic fashion. By the eighteenth century Linnaeus had allocated a Latin binomial (two Latin names) to each plant, in order to distinguish every plant from every other plant. The first name (always with a capital letter) denotes the genus of the plant and the second name (always with a small letter) denotes the species. Latin binomials have now become universal and are the easiest way to avoid confusion, since the common or ordinary name for each plant varies according to region. Even within a small area there are often many different names for the same plant. For example, agrimony is also known as church steeples, cocklebur, sticklewort and philanthropos. And these are just the names it is known by in Britain. So I have used the Latin binomial in addition to the common name of each plant.

When using plants as medicine it is extremely important to use the right plant. I cannot stress this enough. The plant kingdom is full of poisonous plants, many of which are similar to the plants we use as medicine. Some of the plants in this book are so common that most people will have no difficulty identifying them: raspberry and rose for example. However, for the sake of those people who are never quite sure what the difference is between a dandelion and a hawkbit, I shall give a botanical description. Of course there will always be those poor unfortunate souls who, however hard they try, will never be able to identify the right plant, unless it has a label attached to it. For these people I can only advise obtaining the relevant seeds or plants from a reputable herb supplier.

Finding the Herbs

Some of the plants in this book, such as sphagnum moss only grow in very specific places, or appear at particular times of the year, so I have included a description of the plant's habitat and its growing season. You may not be able to find all the herbs anywhere near where you live so again you may need to order seeds from a herb supplier if you wish to grow them.

Growing the Herbs

Each plant requires specific growing conditions. So I have included instructions for growing those that can be cultivated. Some, such as sphagnum moss and watercress require very specific conditions which you may not be able to provide.

Preserving the Herbs

There are many different ways of preserving each herb and the method you choose will depend on the space you have available, whether you can obtain pure (or almost pure) alcohol and what you want to use the herb for. Different methods of preservation determine which healing components will be in the medicine. Different compounds are more, or less, soluble in water, alcohol or fat.

Fresh Herbs

The fresh herb is probably the best way to use leaves and flowers because you will have the benefit of all the healing properties of the plant, whereas the dried herb loses a lot. Volatile oils evaporate to some extent and many other compounds degrade or change in some way.

Fresh Juices

The next best thing to the fresh plant is the fresh juice of the plant. You can buy fresh juices, sealed in airtight bottles for immediate consumption. They can be stored until opened, then kept in the fridge for a few days. Barks and roots don't usually need to be used fresh. They can be dried, ground up or chopped, stewed or extracted with alcohol.

Infusions

Infusions are stronger than herb teas. To make an infusion take one ounce (30g) of dried herb or three ounces (90g) of fresh herb and add one pint of boiling water. Cover and leave to steep for ten minutes. You can make infusions in a tea pot, thermos flask, or any other container with a lid, provided that it is either ceramic, glass or stainless steel. This is the standard dose for most herbal infusions. Water dissolves carbohydrates, peptides, glycosides and tannins.

Decoctions

To make a decoction boil the plant material for one hour, then strain. Make roots, bark and seeds into decoctions.

Teas and Soups

Teas are weaker than infusions. The ancient Celts added herbs to soups and you can too, for example make a soup in spring from young nettles, potatoes and onions.

Tinctures

Tinctures are alcoholic extracts. The Arabs discovered that they could use a mixture of distilled alcohol and water in order to extract and preserve the healing powers from plants. By a process of trial and error they discovered what proportions of alcohol and water to use to extract the maximum healing power from each plant. We now have chemical knowledge that explains why different proportions of water and alcohol are better for extracting different compounds from plants. Some parts of plants, for example, contain large amounts of resin, and to extract this you need almost one hundred per cent alcohol. Herbalists usually leave the chopped plant material to steep for three weeks in the alcohol/water mixture. But if small amounts are ground up more finely, for example in a coffee grinder, twenty-four hours is sufficient, especially if the mixture is shaken at regular intervals. These are the proportions of alcohol and water that are used to extract different types of compounds from plants:

Alcohol Water

90%:10% for resins
60-70%:30-40% for volatile oils
45%:55% for saponins, sterols and most alkaloids
25%:75% for carbohydrates, tannins, peptides, glycosides (which are all water-soluble).

You can make tinctures using wine, if you are extracting plants high in water soluble compounds.

The disadvantage of alcoholic tinctures is that alcohol precipitates proteins and high molecular weight polysaccharides. Therefore alcoholic tinctures are not appropriate for those medicinal plants whose healing properties depend on these compounds. However, the advantage of alcoholic tinctures is that alcohol is a good preserving agent.

Oils

Herbal oils can be made:

(i) By heating the herb in a saucepan with oil. You can use sunflower, olive or corn oil etc. Put as much plant material in the oil as possible and squash it down. Heat without boiling and as the plant material shrinks, add more. Keep adding more until you can't add any more. Heat for about one hour. To make it even stronger, strain off and use the resultant oil to add more herb to.

(ii) By adding the herb to cold oil in a glass container and leaving in the sun to infuse. This is the technique you can use to make calendula oil and hypericum oil, either using the petals or the whole flowers.

Ointments

Some plant constituents are soluble in fats, so this is the best way to extract them. Then they can be kept as an ointment for external use. The Physicians of Myddvai extracted herbs into fats, such as lard, sheep fat, beef fat and butter. All the wound-healing herbs can be made into ointments. Most people today would prefer not to use animal fats to make ointments, but there are several vegetable hard fats, such as cocoa butter and coconut fat. To make an ointment using a hard fat melt the fat in a saucepan and heat the herb in it in the same way as you would do for making a herbal oil, strain, add a few drops of essential oil and pour into jars or pots.

Alternatively you can make an ointment from an oil infusion by heating half a pint of infused oil with a quarter of an ounce of beeswax until the beeswax is dissolved. Stir well and add five drops of lavender or citrus oil to each thirty ounce jar of ointment to preserve it. Benzoin (if you can get it) will also preserve an ointment.

Creams

Some people prefer creams to ointments. These are made by heating thirty grams of beeswax with one hundred millilitres of oil, and then adding one hundred millilitres of herbal infusion with two grams of borax dissolved in it. Pour into jars or pots and add a few drops of essential oil into each container. I have never had much success making creams so I stick to making ointments, which never fail.

Essential Oils

Essential oils are different from ordinary oils. They evaporate at low temperatures and you can extract them by distilling the plant. This is a very expensive and un-ecological way of using plants. Commercially this is done using vast quantities: hundreds of acres of plant material to distil small amounts of essential oil.

Poultices

Poultices work in the same way as ointments. But instead of using fats or oils to absorb the healing principals of the herbs, you can use the whole herb, soaked briefly in hot water and applied externally to the skin of the affected part. The healing principals are absorbed through the skin. This method was popular in ancient times but not so popular today because it is messy and time-consuming. But it is the best way to apply comfrey leaves.

Steam Inhalation

The best way to reach a blocked nose or sinuses is through steam inhalation. Fill a large bowl with very hot water and drop the aromatic herbs onto the surface. Cover your head with a towel, hold it over the bowl and breathe in. Essential oils evaporate off the surface of the hot water and go straight to the affected part.

Fumigation

There are many references to fumigation in the Physicians of Myddvai. They believed that sickness was carried in the air, so they burnt medicinal plants to purify it. This was and is a universal space clearing practice, still used by native people, for example Native Americans, who burn American sage. The sweet smells rise up to the gods, forming a connecting link between the people below and the spiritual realms above. One of the largest parts of the brain is involved with our sense of smell. It connects to our most instinctual part. It also has powerful connections with memory and the unconscious. Powerful smells can be used in ritual, together with music, drumming, and other shamanic practices, to enter into that realm beyond the conscious, which we cannot normally see or hear, and where we find the answers to our urgent questions. Powerful smells, such as incense, are used all over the world to evoke meditative states during religious ceremonies.

Syrup

You can make syrups out of berries, such as rose hips, flowers, such as roses and sometimes even leaves. To make a syrup out of berries simmer five pounds of them with one pound of sugar until it thickens, then strain through a muslin cloth, heat the resultant syrup up again and pour into heated bottles.

Treacle

The word treacle, or triacle, as it was then known, was first used to describe a medical compound called Theriaca Andromachi, or Venice treacle. Theriaca Andromachi, according to Webster's Unabridged Dictionary of 1913 was 'an ancient composition esteemed efficacious against the effects of poison; especially a certain compound of sixty four drugs, prepared, pulverised, and reduced by means of honey to an electuary'. Andromachus was a Greek physician to the Roman Emperor Nero. He apparently invented the famous poison antidote, which would have been very useful in ancient Rome where emperors were constantly in fear of being poisoned. Theriaca is a Greek word, meaning drugs used against the bite of poisonous or wild animals. The word treacle, first used to describe Andromachi's mixture, was later used to describe any remedy which was ground up and mixed with honey. Herbalists in other parts of the world still use this technique and there is no reason why you should not attempt to make your own treacle or electuary, if you have the time and patience.

Choosing the Method of Preservation

I have included methods of preservation for each plant. The methods you choose will depend on the space and time you have available but I would like to invite you to experiment and have fun, perhaps together with like-minded friends.

Chapter 3

Medicinal Plants in the US and the UK

What do we mean when we talk about American medicinal plants and British medicinal plants? Is there a difference? Was there a difference in the past? Is there a difference today?

In the past, before the British settlers came to America, the medicinal plants growing there were, in many cases, different from those growing in Britain. Medicinal herbs, such as Echinacea, *Echinacea purpurea*, golden seal, *Hydrastis canadensis*, American ginseng, *Panax quinquifolius*, black cohosh, *Cimifuga racemosa*, Cascara, *Cascara sagrada* and passion flower, *Passiflora incarnata*, were native to America. Native Americans used these plants as medicine but the early settlers didn't recognise them. They took medicinal herb seeds such as marshmallow, from Britain, planted them and continued to use them. The seeds grew into plants, which produced seeds that blew away and planted themselves. And so these British herbs became American weeds, growing throughout the length and breadth of the continent. Thousands of medicinal plants have made their way to North America, where they have, like the people who brought them, become naturalised.

In some cases the same species of plants, such as Juniper, grew naturally in both Britain and North America, while in other cases although the same genus of plant grew on both sides of the Atlantic, different species grew in Britain and in the US. For example: *Agrimonia eupatoria* or common Agrimony is the most prevalent species of Agrimony in Europe while *Agrimonia gryposepala*, or hairy Agrimony is the most prevalent in North America. Many of the plants used traditionally as medicine in Britain at that time, did not grow in the US. Over time, however, the settlers began using the native American medicinal plants, which later crossed the Atlantic to Europe. Today people in Britain grow American herbs, such as echinacea and black cohosh in their gardens as ornamental plants, while British herb growers cultivate these plants to be sold as tinctures, dried herbs and tablets. On the whole today we grow and use the same herbs in Britain as in the US. The British import herbs from the US and the rest of the world while the US import herbs from all over the world, including Britain.

Part II: The Native Herbs

Chapter 1

Betony *Stachys betonica*

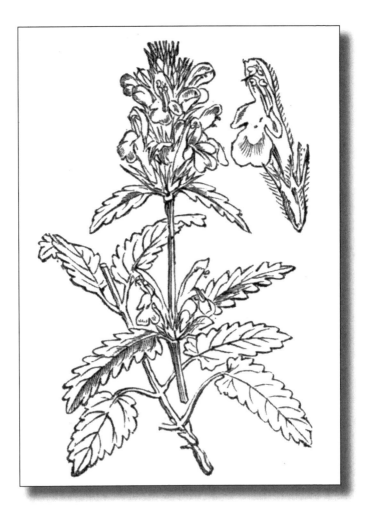

I saw betony for the first time growing in an old meadow in Shropshire when I went to visit my friend Polly. She took me down an ancient lane with steep sides, trees meeting overhead, enclosing it in a leafy tunnel. We climbed out of the lane into a wild meadow surrounded by woodland, with brambles threatening to encroach from the sides. A multitude of different grasses and other plants filled the meadow, wildly competing with each other, stretching up to the sun in all their varying lengths. In amongst this fabulous profusion was betony, with its distinctive dark green leaves. I was excited to find this ancient, Celtic plant that was once so common in Britain and now so rare.

There are five species of *Stachys* growing in Britain, of which *Stachys betonica*, wood betony, is the medicinal one. It was sacred to the Druids and grows in old meadows, open grassland and woodland. According to Mrs Grieve the name Betony derives from the Celtic bew (head) and ton (good), since people believed that it would cure headaches. *Stachys* is Greek, meaning spike, since betony flowers form spikes. The Physicians of Myddvai's book is peppered with references to betony which they used to treat many different symptoms. They believed that it would cure almost everything, including damage from evil spirits, and recommended a mixture of betony juice with wine, honey and nine peppercorns to be drunk morning and evening for nine days for a headache. People sometimes hung the herb round their necks as a protective amulet or charm to guard against evil spirits. Again, according to Mrs Grieve: 'Erasmus said that it would prevent "fearful visions" and "drive away devils and despair".'

It was the most beloved of the bewitching herbs and was used to bathe children who were possessed since the bathwater washed away the bad magic. According to witchepedia some people add betony to protective mixtures, grow it around their homes to protect them or carry it to protect against negativity.

Botanical Description

Betony is perennial with a thickish, woody root. It has straight, square, furrowed stems, one to two feet tall with oblong, stalkless leaves two to three inches long, narrow with indented margins. The majority of the leaves grow from the root and these are larger, on long stalks and an elongated heart shape. All the leaves are rough to the touch and fringed with short, fine hairs; their surface is dotted with glands containing a bitter aromatic oil. The purplish-red, two-lipped flowers grow at the top of stems, arranged in dense rings or whorls, in short spikes. Then there is a break and a piece of bare stem, with two or four oblong stalkless leaves and then more flowers, the whole forming what is termed an interrupted spike, a characteristic unique to wood betony, distinguishing it from all other flowers that belong to the Lamiacae family. Each flower has five sharply pointed sepals and the petals form a long tube ending in two lips, the upper lip slightly arched, the lower one flat, of three equal lobes. There are two pairs of stamens in the arch of the upper lip, one pair longer than the other. The stamens drop pollen on to the backs of the bees who come to drink the honey in the tube, so fertilising the next flower they visit. After fertilisation, four brown, smooth three-cornered seeds develop.

Habitat

Betony is long lived and slow growing, so you tend to find it in old meadows; it prefers short grass on infertile soils. On grasslands that are uncut it eventually loses out to tall, more dominant species. It is no longer common in Britain.

Season

Betony flowers in July and August.

How to Grow

Betony likes damp, slightly acidic soil. Sow the seeds in late summer or autumn because they need to be slightly chilled over the winter to break dormancy.

Parts Used

The whole herb, harvested in July.

Preservation

Choose a nice sunny day to pick your betony and harvest it in the morning, after the dew has evaporated. Cut the stems just above the root, strip off all discoloured or insect-eaten leaves and tie the stalks together, about six per bunch, spread them out fanwise, so that the air can penetrate and hang them over strings to dry in a warm airy place away from the sun. It is important to dry the herbs quickly in order to retain all the healing properties. Store in airtight jars or tins as soon as they are dry.

Properties

Betony is bitter, aromatic, calming and a tonic for the nervous and digestive systems. The British Herbal Pharmacopoeia states that betony is sedative, bitter and good for headache and chronic fatigue syndrome, anxiety, neuralgia and vertigo, frayed nerves, PMS, menopausal depression and panic attacks, taken together with *Scutellaria lateriflora* and *Valeriana officinalis*.

Chemical Constituents

Skaltsa and his team reported that tannins and glycosides were the active components of betony. It also contains betulinic acid, D-camphor, hyperoside, manganese, oleanolic acid, rosmarinic acid, rutin, ursolic acid and stachydrine. There has not been much research into the chemistry of betony. Haznagy-Radnai isolated several anti-inflammatory iridoids, including aucubin and harpagoside.

Research

Very few scientists have thought it worthwhile to carry out research into the healing properties of betony. However, there have been a few trials using other *Stachys* species. In 1974 Peleshchuk gave stachyglen (an extract of flavonoids from *Stachys neglecta*) to eighty-three patients suffering from inflammation of the gall bladder and cholangitis (infection and obstruction of the bile duct). It stimulated the gall bladder to secrete more bile. In 2003 Stamatis found that *Stachys alopecuros* inhibited the bacterium, *Helicobacter pylori, in vitro.* Also in 2003 Rabbani and his team demonstrated that an extract of *Stachys lavandulifolia* stopped rats from being anxious. In the same year Skaltsa tested the volatile oils of eight species of *Stachys* on six types of bacteria and five types of fungi. *Stachys scardica* was the most effective.

In 2006 Matkowski and Piotrowska found that betony was powerfully antioxidant. Then in 2012 Haznagy-Radnai and her team demonstrated that *Stachys officinalis* (betony) was highly anti-inflammatory. They isolated several iridoids and found that the iridoids, aucubin and harpagoside were the most powerfully anti-inflammatory.

How to Use

Catherine Schofield, herbalist, recommends betony's antispasmodic action, which she says makes it an ideal herb for headaches. It will also increase circulation to the brain, thus improving memory. It's a mild tonic, that helps the body to heal itself, slowly, a herb to take over a long period of time since its actions are accumulative. It has an uplifting effect on the mind and spirits over time and is a true brain tonic, protecting the ageing brain against decline. Take an infusion of the dried herb as a tonic and to treat headache, anxiety, depression and chronic fatigue syndrome but do not expect immediate results. It will gradually improve these symptoms. Its antispasmodic effect also calms and strengthens the digestive system so herbalists recommend that people suffering from dyspepsia, weak digestion, nausea, heartburn, colic or irritable bowel syndrome should take an infusion on a regular basis until their symptoms improve.

Dose

Make an infusion with 30g of dried herb and a pint of boiling water and divide this into three portions to drink three times a

day
    2-4 ml liquid extract
    2-6 ml tincture 1:5 45%

Contraindications

Betony appears to be completely safe, except during pregnancy, as it is a mild uterine stimulant.

Chapter 2

Chickweed *Stellaria media*

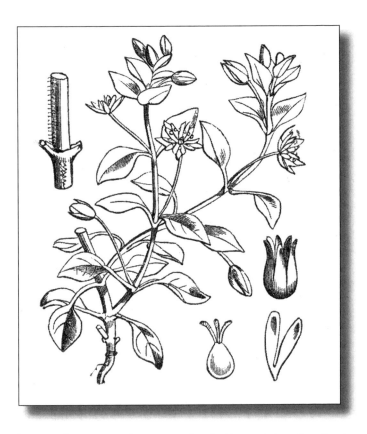

I used to work as an assistant to a herbalist, mixing the tinctures for his patients from the rows of brown bottles in the dispensary. There were little glass pots of comfrey, plantain and chickweed ointments, the three most effective ointments in the dispensary.

Native to all temperate regions, chickweed was growing in Britain at the time of the ancient Celts and since the Physicians of Myddvai used it, this probably indicates that it had been used as a healing herb since ancient times. It has naturalised itself wherever the white man has settled, becoming one of the commonest weeds in North America. Country people in Britain used to add chickweed to salads or boil it and eat it like spinach. Dioscorides (CE 40-90) wrote: 'Alsine, some call it Mouse ear ... from ye having leaves like to ye little ears of a mouse, and it is called Alsine because it loves shady and woody places.' The name Stellaria is from the Latin 'stella' a star, or 'stellaris', starry, because the flowers are shaped like stars and 'media' means medium sized. It was called chickweed because people used to feed it to chicks. Gerard wrote, 'Little birds in cadges are refreshed with the lesser chickweed when they lath their meat.'

Botanical Description

Chickweed spreads out its branching stems as it creeps along the ground. It is juicy, pale green and slightly swollen at the joints. A line of hairs runs up one side of the stem and when it reaches a pair of leaves it continues on the opposite side. The leaves grow in pairs on the stem and are succulent, egg-shaped, about half an inch long and a quarter of an inch broad, with a short point, pale green and smooth, with flat stalks below, but stalkless above. The small white star-like flowers grow singly in the axils of the upper leaves. Their petals are narrow and deeply cleft, and no longer than the sepals. They open about nine o'clock in the morning and remain open for twelve hours in bright weather. But rain prevents them opening, and after a heavy shower they droop downwards instead of turning up towards the sun, though in the course of a few days they open again. The seeds are in a little capsule with teeth, which opens when they are ripe, but close in wet weather. The wind shakes the ripe seeds out of the capsule. Every night the leaves close over the tender buds of the new shoots, and the uppermost pair but one of the leaves at the end of the stalk have longer leaf-stalks than the others, so that they can close over the end pair and protect the tip of the shoot.

Habitat

Chickweed likes ground that has been recently dug or ploughed, but it grows in woodlands, croplands, fallow fields, lawns and gardens, nursery plots, roadsides, shingle riverbanks, coastal cliffs and waste areas. It especially seems to like my allotment.

Season

The flowers appear in March and continue until late autumn.

How to Grow

Chickweed likes a nice fertile soil and a sunny position. It will bloom for one or two months, then set seed and within a short time new plants will spring up. A succession of plants will grow throughout most of the year if you allow them to.

Parts Used

The whole herb, apart from the root.

Preservation

Pick young chickweed plants between May and July and dry it in a warm, airy room.

To make chickweed ointment, dry the chickweed first, then crumble it and add it to sunflower seed or corn oil and heat in a double boiler for one hour without boiling. Strain and add one ounce of beeswax to five ounces of chickweed oil, stir well until the wax is melted and mixed, add a few drops of essential oil of lavender and store the ointment in glass pots.

Properties

Chickweed is anti-rheumatic, anti-inflammatory, astringent, cooling, soothing, emollient, vulnerary and stops itching, according to Khare in 2007, Shinwari in 2000 and Hoffmann in 2003.

Chemical Constituents

Chickweed contains phenolic acids: vanillic, ferulic, caffeic and chlorogenic acids; flavonoids: apigenin, genistein; fatty esters, triterpenoids saponins: gypsogenin; glycosides, anthocynidine, vitamin C, carotene, mucilage and lipids. The leaves are rich in potassium and silicon. Most of the chemical research has been carried out in China and India. In 2005 Hu and his team isolated a number of amino acids from chickweed, including uracil, thymine, thymidine. In the same year Chen isolated apigenin, quercetin and daucosterol from chickweed. In 2007 Huang isolated plant sterols: β-sitosterol, daucosterol, as well as emodin, physcion, questin, 1-hexacosanol, kaempferol-3, 7-O-α-L-dirhamnoside from chickweed. In 2009 Hu isolated a new triterpenoid, together with two known flavonoids, from *Stellaria media* (L.)

Research

Chickweed is a member of the Caryophylaceae family, a plant family that is rich in medicinal plants, particularly those used in China. Plants in this family have anticancer, antibacterial, anti fungal, antiviral, antioxidant and anti-inflammatory properties, according to Chandra in 2015. Major chemical constituents of the Caryophylceae are saponins, phytoecdysteroids, benzenoids, phenyl propanoids and nitrogen containing compounds. In 2011 Chidrawar and his team found that chickweed extracts prevented mice from becoming overweight. They thought that this was due to saponins, flavonoids and beta-sitosterols in the plant.

How to Use

The, anti-inflammatory, astringent, cooling, soothing properties of chickweed make it an ideal ointment to soothe inflammation, burns and skin irritations, such as psoriasis and eczema and draw out infection from wounds. It is also diuretic, expectorant and anti-asthmatic. Make an infusion to soothe coughs, colds and sore throats. Make a tincture with fresh, chopped chickweed and vodka. Shake every day for six weeks, then strain and store in a glass container away from the light. Make a poultice out of fresh chickweed, crushed and applied directly to an inflammation. It will kill bacteria and soothe the inflammation. According to Susan Weed chickweed tincture will cure ovarian cysts. Her evidence is anecdotal but since chickweed contains anti-cancer compounds and plant sterols, it is possible that it could have this effect.

Dose
One ounce of dried herb in two pints of boiling water. Cover and leave to steep for four hours then strain and drink throughout the day.

5 ml of tincture three times a day.

Contraindications
Stellaria media is fatal to lambs and horses if eaten in large quantities. It could cause a temporary form of paralysis in humans if eaten in very large doses. Some people are allergic to chickweed. Pregnant and breastfeeding women should not eat chickweed.

Chapter 3

Horsetail *Equisetum arvense*

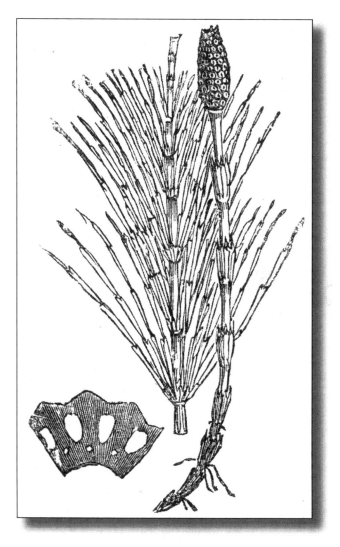

Three years ago I took over an allotment full of weeds. I was determined to dig the whole plot over and rid it of the many varieties of weeds that infested it. There were about one million dandelions, which had had time to send their roots down to Australia. There was couch grass matted in clumps, there was bindweed and there was horsetail. I dug and I dug but I never got to the bottom of the horsetail roots. As fast as I dug them up, more horsetail sprang up from the never ending network of roots under the ground. I did eventually quell the various weeds and plant up my allotment but the horsetail still emerges from time to time.

Horsetails are members of the order Equisetales, an ancient type of plant, unlike any other kind of plant in Britain, but distantly allied to the ferns. The Horsetails that grow in the United States, although the same species, are not the same phenotype as the horsetails that grow in Britain. The name Equisetum derives from the Latin *equus*, meaning horse and *seta*, meaning bristle. Horsetail contains large amounts of silica and people used to sell bunches of the stems for polishing metal, according to Mrs Grieve.

Horsetail has been growing in Britain since the last Ice Age and the ancient Celts will almost certainly have known about its healing properties.

Botanical Description

In spring, horsetail plants send up spore-bearing, fruiting stems that look like thin asparagus shoots, about 15-20cm high. These have cone-like catkins on top, consisting of closely packed cells containing spores. The spores are attached to elastic threads, coiled round the spores when moist, but uncoiled when dry. The plant has roots which both tunnel downwards in search of water and creep along sideways underground, forming a network from which stems grow upwards. Once the spore-bearing stems have died, it sends up jointed, brittle, grooved, barren stems, 10-50 cm tall; hollow except at the joints, with air cells in their walls under the grooves. Toothed sheathes stick out sideways at each joint, all the way round the stem, giving the plant the appearance of a green bottle brush. Young horsetails can grow from spores or straight up from the roots. The barren summer fronds have numerous, thin, jointed branches.

Habitat
Horsetail thrives in damp places, beside rivers and canals, in boggy meadows and in my allotment.

Season
The spore-bearing shoots appear in the spring and the barren bushy stems appear in the early summer.

How to Grow
I really don't advise anyone to grow horsetail, since it is impossible to control once it has taken root and will spread everywhere, even breaking through tarmac, appearing in the middle of pavements in Britain in particularly wet years.

Parts Used
The barren stems after the fruiting stems have died down. Cut the barren stems off just above the root. Use fresh or dried.

Preservation
Pick the barren stems and dry them in a warm, airy place away from the sun.

Chemical Constituents
Horsetail contains alkaloids: nicotine, palustrine and palustrinine; and saponins and lignin glycosides. It is rich in vitamins C and E and has high levels of silica, copper and zinc, as well as aluminium, sulphur, magnesium and manganese. It contains phytosterols including cholesterol, campesterol and β-sitosterol, according to Takatsuto in 1992. In 2004 Oh and his team isolated phenolic petrosins from *E arvense*, as

well as flavonoids, including apigenin, luteolin, kaempferol and quercetin. In 2006 Radulovic isolated several volatile oil compounds from *E arvensis*, including thymol.

Research

Several scientists in Japan and China, (including Kuriyama in 1998, who patented anti-acne, anti-sebum, anti-bacterial and anti-dandruff compositions with *E arvense* extracts in them), have patented a wide range of skin and hair products containing horsetail extracts, for use as face creams, soaps, shampoos, hair restorers etc. These patents state that horsetail acts as anti-ageing, moisturiser, anti-wrinkle, anti-acne, antiperspirant, conditioner and that it strengthens and maintains hair tone and prevents grey hair and dandruff.

Scientists have carried out a great deal of research on horsetail, almost all of it in the laboratory. In 1998 Yu and his team found that *E arvense* extracts inhibited HIV *in vitro*. In 2002 Samura found that a mixture of plant extracts, including *Equisetum arvense*, had a calming effect on the nervous system of animals. In 2003 Sakurai and his team found that *E arvensis* relaxed the walls of blood vessels *in vitro*. In 2004 Oh found that onitin and luteolin from *E arvense* protected liver cells *in vitro*, and scavenged free radicals. Also in 2004 Hoffmann Martins do Monte and his team found that an extract of *E arvense* reduced pain and swelling in mice and Hassane and his team found that the juice of the plant helped blood to coagulate. They thought that it might stop stomach ulcers from bleeding and thus prevent anaemia. In 2005 Nagai and his team found that the phenolic part of horsetail extract was a powerful antioxidant and Monte found that *E arvense* extract reversed the cognitive impairment in old rats. In 2006 Radulovic found that the volatile oil compounds in *E arvensis* were powerfully anti-bacterial and anti-candida and Zhang recommended using horsetail for treating haemorrhoids. In 2007 Soleimani and his team found that an extract of *E arvense* had anti-diabetic activity in rats and Alexandru and his team found that *E arvense* extract killed leukaemia cells *in vitro*. In 2008 Canadanovic-Brunet and his team found that extracts of *E arvense* were powerfully anti-bacterial and antioxidant.

In 2014 Carneiro and his team carried out a small clinical trial. Thirty-six healthy men, divided into three groups, took it in turns to take *E arvense* extract, placebo and hydrochlorothiazide (25 mg/day) for four consecutive days. They found that the *E arvense* extract was as powerful a diuretic as hydrochlorothiazide and the men taking it did not become deficient in any essential minerals. It appeared to be safe when taken for a short period, but this was a small trial and further research is needed.

How to Use

Horsetail is diuretic, astringent, anodyne and anti-inflammatory. The high silica content helps wounds, fractures and sprains to heal. It strengthens and regenerates connective tissues. If you make a decoction and use it to wash wounds it will stop them from bleeding. It will also help poorly healing wounds and ulcers to heal. Drink glassfuls of the decoction during menstruation to prevent excessive bleeding and use it to treat nose bleeds and bleeding ulcers. The local astringent and anti-hemorrhagic effect explains why people use horsetail to treat bleeding from the mouth, bleeding haemorrhoids, to check diarrhoea, dysentery and for chilblains and conjunctivitis. People take infusions of horsetail for brittle fingernails and hair loss, gout, swelling and to treat catarrh. It eases the pain of rheumatism and stimulates the healing of chilblains. It improves blood circulation. *Equisetum arvense* is an excellent genito-urinary system astringent. People use it to treat urethritis or cystitis, but if this condition persists you must see a doctor.

Horsetail improves hair condition and will heal most skin conditions, including acne and eczema. It improves the texture and tone of skin, even mature skin or skin that shows signs of premature ageing. Several cosmetics contain horsetail extract, together with UV adsorbents and act as moisturisers and skin conditioning agents. Some people even suggest that horsetail contains a hidden 'youth factor'. The extract is used in shower gel, shampoo, soap and cosmetic cleanser.

Dose

Infusion 2-3 tsp dried horsetail infused for 10 minutes. Drink a cupful 3 times a day.

Contraindications

Do not take horsetail long term, since it could decrease levels of vitamin B1, cause digestive problems, nervous disorders, headaches and loss of appetite. People with heart or kidney disorders, diabetes, or gout should not use horsetail. Do not take during pregnancy or lactation.

Chapter 4

Juniper Berry *Juniperus communis*

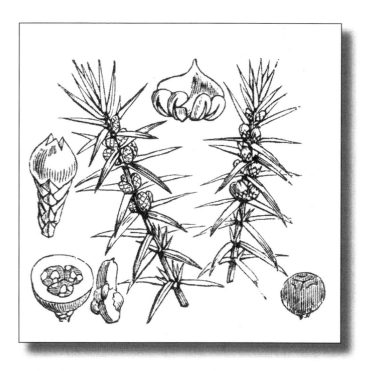

Juniper has been growing in Britain for thousands of years and was probably known to the ancient Celts. People have been distilling the berries for centuries to extract the essential oil. Commercially juniper berries are used to flavour teas, beers, liqueurs (ginepro) alcoholic bitters and gin. The word gin may be a shortened form of the Dutch genever, which is derived from the Latin *juniperus,* or it may be derived from the term Holland's Geneva, as the Dutch-invented drink was first known.

Botanical Description

Juniper is a member of the Cypress family: the Cupressaceae and can grow as a dense, evergreen shrub, creeping along the

47

ground, or a small tree, up to twenty feet high. It has dark green to blue green pointed leaves and blue or reddish berries a quarter to half an inch wide. Juniper berries take two or three years to ripen, so that there are blue and green berries on the same plant.

Habitat
It grows on chalk downs near London, on the limestone hills of the Lake District, on the Scottish mountains and on heath-like, siliceous soils where some lime occurs.

Season
The berries ripen in the autumn.

How to Grow
It is important to grow *Juniperus communis* and not one of the many ornamental varieties of Juniper, which do not have the same medicinal properties. It likes a sunny slope and chalky soil.

Parts Used
The berries.

Preservation
Pick the berries when they are ripe and dry them.

Properties
According to Barnes in 2007, Juniper is anti-rheumatic, antiseptic, carminative, diuretic and stomachic. Juniper oil is astringent, anti-inflammatory and antiseptic.

Chemical Constituents
In 2005 Nakanishi and his team isolated neolignans and flavonoid glycosides from *Juniperus communis*. In 2009 Gordien isolated sequiterpenes and diterpenes. In 2003 Shamir extracted volatile oil from the berries and the needles of *Juniperus communis*.

The needle oil consisted mainly of sabinene (40.7%), α-pinene (12.5%) and terpinen-4-ol (12.3%) and the berry oil included sabinene (36.8%), α-pinene (20%), limonene (10.6%), germacrene D (8.2%) and myrcene (4.8%). Juniper also contains flavonoids, biflavonyls and fatty acids.

Research

There have been some *in vitro* and animal studies on juniper but no one has yet carried out any human clinical studies. Traditionally people have used juniper to treat tuberculosis, so in 2009 Gordien and his team decided to investigate the anti-tuberculosis compounds in it. They isolated and identified a sesquiterpene: longifolene and a diterpene: totarol from *Juniperus communis* roots. They found that these compounds killed antibiotic resistant *Mycobacterium tuberculosis,* one of the bacteria that cause tuberculosis. They isolated another diterpene from the above ground part of the plant: *trans*-communic acid, which killed another bacterium that causes tuberculosis. Unfortunately these compounds also kill human cells. In 2009 Miceli and his team isolated 16 flavonoids from an extract of the berries of *Juniperus communis*. The extract was antioxidant and antibacterial. According to Carroll in 2011 the essential oil from *J. communis* repels ticks and the mosquitoes that transmit yellow fever *in vitro,* almost as powerfully as Deet.

How to Use

Juniper is a very powerful medicine, should be used with great care and never long term. It detoxifies the body, promotes elimination of uric acid and so herbalists use it to treat inflammatory diseases such as gout and rheumatoid arthritis. According to Robbers and Tyler it inhibits the formation of inflammatory prostaglandins. Herbalists combine it with other herbs as a diuretic to treat urinary problems, although the German Commission E does not approve juniper for kidney and bladder complaints. However, in 2008 Health Canada recommended juniper fruit as a diuretic and urinary tract antiseptic to help relieve benign urinary tract infections. They also recommended using it as a carminative to help relieve digestive disturbances, such as flatulent dyspepsia, to aid digestion and stimulate appetite. The German Commission E does approve aqueous infusions and decoctions of juniper dried fruit, alcoholic extracts, wine extracts or essential oil to relieve indigestion or disturbed digestion. In addition juniper berries help clear congestion and are often included in cold remedies to improve breathing.

Massage with the diluted essential oil eases neuralgia, sciatica and rheumatic pains. According to Mrs Grieve, Juniper oil is good for indigestion, flatulence, heartburn, bloating, loss of appetite, gastrointestinal infections, intestinal worms and diseases of the kidney and bladder. Juniper oil helps to cleanse and tone the skin in cases of skin inflammations such as acne and eczema. Juniper oil has a strengthening, tonic effect on the nerves. You can inhale the essential oil of juniper to treat bronchitis.

Dose

Infusion of 1 oz (30 g) of the berry to 1 pint of boiling water every twenty-four hours. 1:1 liquid extract with 25% ethanol, and 1:5 tincture with 45% ethanol: 0.1 ml. 20 to 100 mg of the essential oil diluted in a carrier oil for massage.

Contraindications

Juniper is the most active but also the most potentially toxic of the volatile-oil-containing berries used to treat infections of the urinary tract according to Robbers and Tyler. Use Juniper with great care and do not take on a regular basis. Do not use during pregnancy or lactation or where there is kidney disease. Overdose can cause convulsions and damage the kidneys. Use juniper berry essential oils sparingly. Some people are allergic to juniper.

Chapter 5

Marshmallow *Althea officinalis*

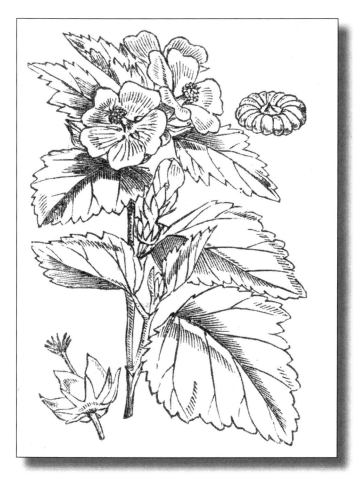

According to Harry Godwin, *Althea officinalis* has been growing in Britain for many thousands of years and Seddon found plenty of its pollen in the lower layers of peat at Avonmouth on the Bristol Channel in 1965. Gerard mentions that marshmallow, 'groweth very plentifully in the marshes both on the Kentish and Essex shore alongst the river of Thames, about Woolwich, Erith,

Greenhyth, Gravesend, Tilburie, Lee, Colchester, Harwich and in most salt marshes about London.' However, today Marshmallow is listed as nationally scarce in Britain and it is forbidden to collect it in the wild.

The Greek name *'althaia'* is derived from the words *'althos'*: a medicine, *'altho'*: to cure and *'althaiein'*: to heal. According to Mrs Grieve its family name Malvaceae is derived from the Greek *malake*, meaning soft. The Physicians of Myddvai used mallow in many of their remedies which suggests that the ancient Celts knew about it and used it as medicine.

Botanical Description

Althea officinalis has tall, stiff, velvety stems, up to 150 cm high, with velvety leaves growing on alternate sides all the way up the stem. The leaves have three to five shallow lobes, folded like a fan. The flowers are pale pink with five broad petals and grow in clusters all the way up the stem from May to September. It is similar to hollyhock, the old-fashioned garden flower.

Habitat

It is a coastal plant, characteristic of the upper margins of salt marshes.

Season

May to September.

Growing Conditions

Sow the seeds ten to twelve weeks before the last frost in seed trays and keep them moist and cool all the time. Plant them out after the last frost. They will grow in almost any kind of soil.

Parts Used

Dried leaves and dried roots.

Preservation

Dig up the root of two-year-old cultivated plants in the autumn. Do not dig up the wild plants. Collect the leaves just before flowering.

Properties

Everything about this plant is soft: its soft, velvety leaves and stem, its soft, soothing effect on the throat as it slips down, soothing the stomach and the rest of the digestive tract. Marshmallow is a demulcent, or soothing herb, because it contains large amounts of mucilage. The more the dried plant swells in water, the more soothing it will be. Demulcent plants contain polysaccharides, compounds made up of large numbers of sugar molecules joined together in long, branching chains. These compounds expand as they absorb water and form a demulcent gel. In marshmallow the polysaccharides are highly branched and absorb a lot of water to form a mucus-like gel which clings to the surface of mucous membranes, such as the throat, soothing it. Pharmacopeial quality marshmallow root should have a swelling index of not-less-than ten, and for marshmallow leaf, not-less-than twelve, according to the European Pharmacopoeia Commission.

In 1989 the German Commission E approved both marshmallow leaf and root for irritation of the mouth and throat and dry cough. The Commission also approved the root for mild inflammation of the stomach lining. According to Schultz in 1998, since mucilage forms a protective layer on the lining of the throat, it reduces the irritation of receptors, thus soothing a cough. Marshmallow is also expectorant, so particularly good for making a dry irritating cough productive. Demulcents, unlike opioid-based cough suppressants, are neither sedative nor addictive.

It also soothes the digestive system, so has a calming effect on gastritis, gastric or peptic ulceration and enteritis, and specifically for gastric and duodenal ulcer. Marshmallow ointment soothes and softens grazes, cracks, inflammation and insect stings. It also soothes the urinary tract.

Chemical constituents in the root

Marshmallow root contains 11% mucilage, according to Bradley in 1992. This mucilage is composed of Polysaccharides: galacturonic acid, glucuronic acid, rhamnose, arabinose, zylose, mannose, galactose and glucose, according to Blaschek and Franz in 1986. In 1991 Gudej identified a number of phenolic acids, including caffeic, p-coumaric, ferulic, salicylic, vanillin and syringic. It also contains the coumarin: scopoletin, and the flavonoids: glycosides of hypolaetin and isoscutellarein.

Chemical constituents in the leaf

Marshmallow leaf contains 10% mucilage, according to Blaschek and Franz in 2006. This mucilage is composed of Polysaccharides: Rhamnose, glucuronic acid and galacturonic acid, according to Shimizo and Tomoda 1985. In 1990 Gudej identified the flavonoids: tiliroside and glycosides of hypolaetin, quercetin, kaempferol.

Chemical constituents in the flowers

In 1991 Dzido found tiliroside, and the flavones: glycosides of hypolaetin, kaaempferol, dihydrokaempferol in the flowers.

Research

In 2003 Zerehsaz carried out a clinical study on 42 patients in Iran with chronic cutaneous leishmaniasis. Leishmaniasis is caused by the *Leishmania* parasite, which is transmitted by the sandfly. It can take three forms: visceral leishmaniasis, which is often fatal, diffuse cutaneous leishmaniasis, which is hideously disfiguring and cutaneous leishmaniasis, which takes the form of a tropical sore. Zerehsaz applied a paste made up of marshmallow and hollyhock and other herbs to the sores. 69% of the patients recovered completely, 12% were partially cured and 19% did not respond to the treatment. It is a pity that we do not know what all the ingredients in the paste were because this is a significant result for a disease that affects millions of people worldwide, people who are generally poor and can only afford herbal treatments.

Also in 2003 Brinckmann carried out a double-blind, placebo-controlled study on 60 patients in the US with acute pharyngitis (sore throat). He gave half the patients a herbal tea (throat Coat, Traditional Medicinals, Sebastopol CA) that contained marshmallow root, licorice root (*Glycyrrhiza glabra*), slippery elm bark (*Ulmus rubra*) and wild cherry bark (*Prunus serotina*), among others. He gave the other half of the patients a placebo. The tea provided a rapid, temporary relief of sore throat pain that was far superior to the placebo.

In 2005 Buechi carried out a clinical study on 62 patients with irritating cough. He gave them a cough syrup (Weleda Hustenelixier) which contained extracts of ivy leaf, (*Hedera helix*), thyme leaf (*Thymus vulgaris*), wild thyme leaf (*T. serpyllum*), anise fruit (*Pimpinella anisum*) and marshmallow root. The syrup alleviated coughs resulting from common colds, bronchitis and respiratory tract diseases that formed mucous.

In 2007 Sutovska tested a mucilage polysaccharide extract from marshmallow flowers on cats with coughs. It was more effective than the non-narcotic drug dropropizine. However, it was less effective than codeine at reducing the cough but did not have codeine's unfortunate side effect of reducing expectoration.

Also in 2007 scientists in Iran carried out a randomised controlled trial on people with high blood pressure, who had developed a cough as a side effect of their Angiotensin converting enzyme (ACE) inhibitor medication. Sixty-three adults took 40 mg of *Althea officinalis* root, as 20 drops of extract, daily for 4 weeks. At the end of the trial the patients said that their cough was much less severe. This is interesting, as coughing can be a troublesome side effect of this type of medication, which doctors frequently recommend for high blood pressure. It would be a good idea to carry out further research with larger numbers of patients.

How to Use

Add marshmallow tincture to cough mixtures, for its wonderful soothing properties. It will calm the patient and make a dry cough productive. Take a warm infusion of the root, or tincture three times a day, to soothe a dry cough or take a spoonful of the syrup to allay an acute bout of coughing. Take an infusion to soothe colitis, acid indigestion and urinary stones. Rub marshmallow ointment on inflamed skin and joints, ulceration, stings and bites, neuralgia and inflamed breasts.

Preparation

To make an infusion, add 15g of dried marshmallow root to a pint of cold water and leave to macerate overnight. Strain and divide into three equal portions. Drink three times a day.

Make an ointment by grinding up 5 grams of dried root to a fine powder and mixing into a hundred grams of a neutral ointment base.

Dose

Tincture 2-5 ml.
Syrup BPC 1949 2-10 ml.
Infusion 15 g divided into three equal portions.

Contraindications

Marshmallow is safe in pregnancy and lactation. Do not take marshmallow for long periods of time since it could possibly reduce the absorption of other medicines.

Chapter 6

Meadowsweet *Filipendula ulmaria*

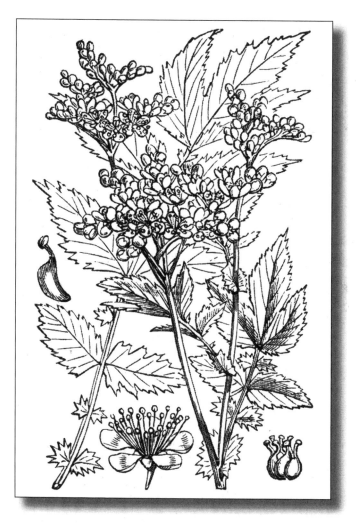

There is something quintessentially British about the sweet perfume of meadowsweet, flowering on riverbanks, beside canals
and in boggy meadows, with its creamy white flowers and feath-
ery leaves. It may not be as common now as it was when I was

a child.

Meadowsweet belongs to the rose family (Rosaceae) and was one of the Druids' sacred herbs, according to Mrs Grieve. The Physicians of Myddvai used it to treat all sorts of conditions, which strongly suggests that the ancient Celts used it as medicine. It is mentioned in Geoffrey Chaucer's Knight's Tale.

Gerard wrote in his Herball, in 1597:

The leaves and floures of Meadowsweet farre excelle all other strowing herbs for to decke up houses, to strewe in chambers, halls and banqueting-houses in the summer-time, for the smell thereof makes the heart merrie and joyful and delighteth the senses.

In mediaeval and Elizabethan times people covered the floors of banqueting halls with sweet smelling strewing herbs, which released their perfume as the guests crushed them with their feet. Meadowsweet was Queen Elizabeth I's favourite strewing herb. Cooks used the herb to flavour beers, meads and wines and added it to soups for an interesting almond flavour. People soaked it in rainwater and used it as an astringent and skin conditioner.

Botanical Description

Meadowsweet has dark green leaves, divided into many pointed leaflets, a few of which are large and tooth edged, with small intermediate ones. The leaves have downy whitish undersides. The leaflets at the end of the stalk are one to three inches long with three to five lobes. The stems, which are sometimes purple, can grow two to four feet high, erect and furrowed. The flowers are small, clustered close together in handsome irregularly-branched combs, and have a very strong, sweet smell of almonds. The leaves are also perfumed.

Habitat

Meadowsweet likes wet places like riverbanks, canals and boggy meadows.

Season

Meadowsweet flowers in June and July. Harvest in July, when in flower.

How to Grow

Meadowsweet needs nice damp soil with plenty of organic material, such as compost, dug in. So if you have a boggy patch in your garden where water tends not to drain away, this is an ideal place to plant meadowsweet.

Parts Used

Leaves and flowers.

Preservation

Cut off the tops of the plants in July and dry them in a warm, airy room away from direct sunlight.

Properties

Filipendula ulmaria's pain killing effect is due to salicylic acid, which is released from various compounds in the plant, such as salicyl-aldehyde and methyl-salicylate as they pass through the digestive system, according to Papp in 2008. Meadowsweet is diaphoretic, anti-inflammatory, astringent, antiseptic and analgesic.

Chemical Constituents

In 1835 the Swiss pharmacist, Pagenstecher extracted salicyl aldehyde from meadow sweet flowers. Meadowsweet contains volatile and non-volatile salicylates, including salicylic acid, a painkiller which unfortunately irritates the stomach. The chemists who first discovered salicylic acid in both meadowsweet and willow bark transformed it into acetylsalicylic acid, the famous drug aspirin, which is less irritant. But meadowsweet also contains phenolic compounds, including ellagitannins, which protect the wall of the stomach and the intestines from the irritating effect of the salicylates. It contains caffeic, coumaric, anisic, gallic, gentisic, ferulic, chlorogenic and vanilic acids; apigenin, rododendrol, esculetin, and m-hydroxybenzoic acids, according to Shilova in 2006; and the flavonoids: quercetin and its glycosides and rutin. It also contains volatile oils, mucilage, coumarin, carbohydrates, vitamin C and vitamin E.

Research

In 1997 Halkes and his team and in 1999 Kähkönen and her team found that extracts of *Filipendula ulmaria* roots, leaves and flowers were antioxidant. In 2001 Calliste and his team demonstrated that *F ulmaria* extracts were not only antioxidant but also stopped melanoma cells from multiplying *in vitro*. Then in 2011 Barros and her team discovered that the antioxidant properties of the plant were due to the phenolic compounds, including tannins, flavonoids and vitamins that it contained. Antioxidants protect our cells from damage due to toxins in the environment and the general wear and tear of daily life. They may help to protect us from cardiovascular disease and certain forms of cancer. In 2014 Lima and his team showed that flower extracts of *F ulmaria* stopped three different types of tumour cells, including melanoma, lung cancer and breast cancer cells, from multiplying *in vitro*.

In 2013 Nitta and his team isolated four ellagitannins from *Filipendula ulmaria* flowers and tested them to see whether they would inhibit histidine decarboxylase (HDC). HDC is necessary for the formation of histamine, which can trigger allergic reactions. The four ellagitannins inhibited HDC, so they acted as anti-histamines.

In 2015 Neagu and her team found that extracts of *F ulmaria* inhibited acetyl-cholineserase. Acetylcholine stimulates several areas in the brain which play important roles in arousal, attention and motivation. Actyl-cholinesterase breaks down acetylcholine. Doctors prescribe pharmaceutical acetyl-cholinesterase inhibitors to stop acetyl-cholinesterase from breaking down acetyl choline, so that it remains in the brain stimulating arousal, attention and motivation. This helps to treat the memory loss and learning symptoms of dementia. So Neagu and her team suggested that since meadowsweet extracts inhibit acetyl-cholineserase, they could be used to treat the symptoms of degenerative diseases such as Alzheimer's and Parkinson's.

In 2009 Boziaris and his team demonstrated that extracts of *F ulmaria* could prevent food-borne bacteria such as salmonella from breeding and multiplying. This was due to the phenolic compounds, such as caffeic, coumaric and vanilic acids, in the extracts. In 2015 Katanic and her team found that extracts of the arial parts and root of *F ulmaria* were antioxidant and anti-bacterial, especially against *E coli* and *E faecalis* and against the fungi *P cyclopium* and *F oxysporum*. The root extract was highly antioxidant. She suggested that these extracts could be used as food preservatives.

Unfortunately few scientists have carried out any clinical trials with meadowsweet, so although we know that it contains many valuable compounds with painkilling, anti-bacterial and anti-oxidant properties, we do not have hard, scientific evidence that it is effective. However, herbalists have been using it to treat many painful conditions for centuries and swear that it works.

How to Use

Since meadowsweet is anti-inflammatory and a painkiller, take an infusion of the flowers to alleviate the pain of inflamed joints, for arthritis, rheumatism, headaches and neuralgia. The tannins and mucilage in it protect the wall of the gut, making it valuable for healing heartburn, gastritis, diarrhoea, enteritis, acid indigestion, peptic ulcers, and gastric ulceration. An infusion will help to relieve intestinal wind. Take meadowsweet infusion for colds, coughs and influenza. It relaxes the muscles and encourages sleep. Since it is gently diuretic it helps to rid the body of toxic wastes and uric acid so since it is also astringent and antiseptic, it helps clear up skin diseases.

Dose

2.5 to 3.5 g/day of dried flowers.

Make a tea from 4-6 g of dried herb and take 3 times daily.

Contraindications

Meadowsweet contains salicylates so it may increase the risk of bleeding when the patient is taking anticoagulant or non-steroidal anti-inflammatory drugs (NSAIDs), or any anti-platelet medicines. Patients with salicylate or sulphite sensitivity should not use meadowsweet. Patients with asthma should use it with caution. Pregnant and lactating women should not take it. According to the American Gastroenterological Association (AGA), each year the side effects of NSAIDs hospitalise over 100,000 people and kill 16,500 people in the US alone. The most common side effects of aspirin include bleeding ulcers and tinnitus. Ironically, meadowsweet is commonly used by herbalists to heal the problems which aspirin creates. By isolating salicin from meadowsweet and willow and turning it into aspirin, the pharmaceutical industry has left out natural buffering agents found in the whole plant.

Chapter 7

Mugwort *Artemisia vulgaris*

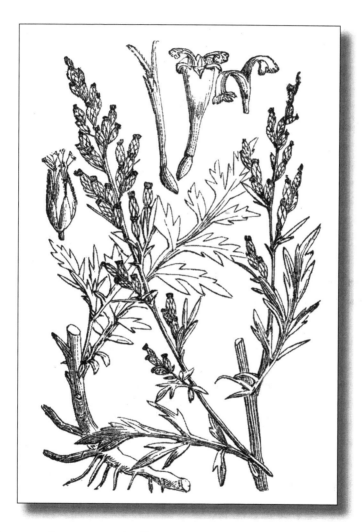

Mugwort has grown in Britain since ancient times and was much loved by the Physicians of Myddvai, so was almost certainly used by the ancient Celts. Pliny said that the Latin name Artemisia derived from the Greek goddess, Artemis, since the herb is particularly good for curing women's diseases. As soon as Artemis was born she helped to deliver her twin, Apollo the sun god. So she became the goddess of childbirth, although she never married or had any children of her own. Artemis is queen of the witches, Goddess of the moon, herbalist, midwife, birthing woman and hunter. She is an untamed, wild woman who runs free with the deer, the wolves and the hounds. Her name was given to various members of the *Artemisia* genus because of their action on the female womb and menstrual cycle, according to O'Dowd in 2001. Pliny also said Artemisia was named after Artemisia the Second, wife of Mausolus, ruler of Caria 377-353 BCE, a land in Asia minor now an area of southwest Turkey. Artemisia the Second was renowned for her extraordinary grief at the death of her husband, entertaining no new husband but pining away until her death two years later. She built a majestic burial tomb to her husband at Halicarnassus, which was considered one of the Seven Wonders of the World. The ruins of this mausoleum are in modern Bodrum.

In many ancient cultures mugwort was considered a magical plant, to be worn or held by people who desired clairvoyant powers and the ability to see clearly, according to *A Women's Book of Herbs* by Brooke. The Salernitan Herbal says mugwort was used to stop bad thoughts and frighten away devils. It is a magical herb of the moon goddess, according to Corinna Wood. Like the moon, mugwort invites us to travel with her from the material world into the magical. Susan Weed says that over the growing season this plant will transition from a plant that nurtures our bodies into one that feeds our souls. Pliny said that it protects a person who carries it on his person from witchcraft and sorcery, poison and venomous beasts, particularly toads, and will prevent a traveller from feeling fatigue on his journey. People used to wear garlands of mugwort on St John's Eve as they danced around the midsummer fire, then throw them into the fire to cast off misfortune, so the plant is called St John's crown. The Physicians of Myddvai suggest taking an eggshell full of the juice of mugwort and garlic in the morning before a long journey to ensure that the person would come to no harm. Nor would they feel tired during the journey, however far they walked.

Mugwort is closely related to the desert sage (*Artemisia tridentate*) which the Pueblo people of New Mexico burn as a smudge to cleanse their dwellings and prepare a sacred space for ritual. It is also related to wormwood (*Artemisia absinthium*) which is in the narcotic liqueur absinthe, much loved by Toulouse-Lautrec.

Botanical Description
Mugwort has ribbed, reddish stems, 50-180 cm high. Pointed leaves grow out of alternate sides of the stem, smooth and green on the upper side and white and downy underneath. Lower leaves have stalks and are divided into many pointed lobes, upper leaves have no stalks and are long, thin and pointed, like spears. From July to September mugwort produces dense, tapering panicles of inconspicuous, oval, rayless, reddish flower-heads.

Habitat
It tends to grow in waste places and disturbed ground, where it can form dense clumps.

Season
Mugwort flowers from July to September.

How to Grow
Mugwort grows best in a sunny place but it's not fussy about the kind of soil it grows in, although it will grow better if you dig in lots of compost. Plant the seeds in the autumn. If you let your plants go to seed they will multiply quickly so you will need to dig them up if they threaten to take over the garden.

Preservation

Mugwort grows well over four feet high so only pick the most vibrant upper parts and leave the dry lower one or two feet. Pick the flowering tops of mugwort as soon as they come into flower and hang them up to dry in a warm airy place away from direct sunlight.

Properties

Mugwort is a real woman's herb that stimulates menstrual flow and normalises and tones the reproductive system. It is an emmenogogue: i.e., it stimulates menstrual flow and brings on the menses when the patient is suffering from delayed menstruation, amenorrhoea, (no menstruation at all) dysmenorrhoea (irregular menstruation) and pre-menstrual syndrome. The National Herbal Pharmacopoeia suggests using it for painful or irregular menstruation and amenorrhoea. In ancient times emmenogogues were used as abortifacients and the large number of such herbs mentioned in the Physicians of Myddvai shows just how important this was before the age of modern contraception.

Mugwort is also a bitter tonic for the digestive system. The British Herbal Pharmacopoeia recommends using it to treat poor appetite, nervous indigestion and intestinal worms. The National Botanic Pharmacopoeia says mugwort is diaphoretic and restores the nervous system. Herbalists today use mugwort to tone the nervous system, ease depression and tension. It comforts the grieving, removes irritability and eases painful joints in the elderly. Several of the ancient herbalists recommended mugwort for breaking up kidney stones, but no research has been carried out to prove or disprove this.

Chemical Constituents

Mugwort has 0.2-0.4% volatile oil according to Judzentiene and Buzelyte in 2006. This includes sabinene, alpha-pinene, 1 8-cineole, alpha-thujone, beta-thujone, germacrene D, carophyllene, mycene, vulgarole, camphor and camphene. Nano and his team in Italy found that the concentrations of these volatile oil compounds varied with time of year and were higher during flowering. Bahorun identified flavonoids, including apigenin, quercetin, kaempferol and isorhamnetin. In 2003 Fraisse identified chlorogenic acid and dicaffeoylquinic acid from the flowering tops. In 1998 Lee identified the flavones: luteolin, eriodictyol, vitexin, apigenin and flavone methylethers. Murray and Stefanovic identified the coumarin, dracunculin in 1986.

Research
There has been very little research into the healing properties of mugwort, apart from the identification of some of its constituents.

How to Use
Make an infusion of the flowering tops for painful, irregular or delayed menstruation, amenorrhoea, and pre-menstrual syndrome, to tone the whole reproductive system and stimulate menstrual flow. Drink mugwort tea when you are feeling depressed or suffering from premenstrual nervous tension and irritability. It will calm you and restore your mood. Make an infusion when you have no appetite and your stomach and digestive system are feeling upset and irritable. It will stimulate your appetite and calm your digestion. Take mugwort tincture, mugwort vinegar or tea to tone and improve the urinary, digestive, hormonal, nervous and circulatory systems. Make a dream pillow from the dried leaves of mugwort to stimulate vivid and creative dreams.

Dose
1 oz (30 g) of fresh herb to 1 pint of boiling water, left to steep, then taken in wineglassful doses (3-4 tablespoons or 45-60 ml) three times a day.

500 mg-2g dried herb three times a day.

0.5 ml tincture three times a day.

Contraindications

Do not use during pregnancy or lactation. Do not use if the patient is allergic to mugwort or any other members of the plant family Asteraceae, or if they are allergic to birch, celery, hazelnut, kiwi fruit or peach. Mugwort pollen is a common aero-allergen. Do not use to prevent malaria. Travellers who took mugwort to prevent malaria when they travelled to Africa, caught malaria. There has been a great deal of publicity around the discovery that the Chinese plant, *Artemisia annua* is an effective antimalarial. However, mugwort does not contain artemisenin, the active compound in *Artemisia annua*, and in any case even if it did artemisenin has a short half life and is therefore not useful for prophylaxis. In 2005 Kurtzhals tested mugwort on the malaria parasite *in vitro* and showed that it had no effect.

Chapter 8

Great Mullein *Verbascum thapsus*

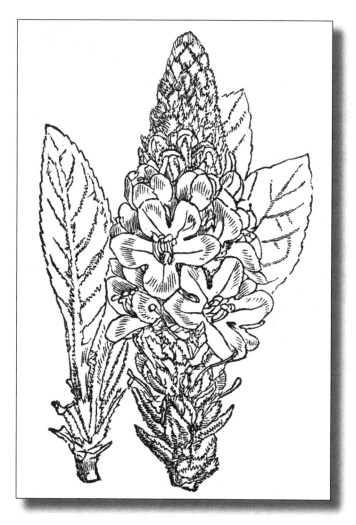

Great mullein is an ancient plant that used to be a common sight in hedgerows in Britain. Linnaeus gave it its Latin name *Verbascum,* which may be a corruption of *barbascum,* from the Latin *barba* (a beard), because of its hairy leaves. Centuries ago people used to dry the down on the leaves and stem to use as tinder, since it would ignite with the slightest spark and they called it 'Candlewick Plant' because they used it for lamp wicks. Some people called it 'Hag's Taper' because they believed that witches used lamps and candles with mullein-down wicks, as they chanted their incantations. But the word 'hag' may have derived from the Anglo-Saxon word *Haege* or *Hage* (a hedge). Great mullein was also called 'Hedge Taper' and 'Our Lady's Candle,' possibly because it looked like a candle growing in the hedge.

Lyte tells us that: 'the whole toppe, with its pleasant yellow floures sheweth like to a wax candle or taper cunningly wrought.' 'Torches' is another name for the plant, and Parkinson tells us:

'*Verbascum* is called of the Latines *Candela regia*, and *Candelaria*, because the elder age used the stalks dipped in suet to burne, whether at funeralls or otherwise.' Coles says that: 'Husbandmen of Kent do give it their cattle against the cough of the lungs, and I, therefore, mention it because cattle are also in some sort to be provided for in their diseases.'

People used to believe that mullein would drive away evil spirits. Ulysses took Mullein with him to protect himself against the wiles of Circe.

Botanical Description

Great mullein, a member of the Scrophulariaceae family, is a tall biennial with a thick stem, which frequently grows up to four or five feet high in the wild and can even reach seven or eight feet in gardens. It has large leaves and flowers in long, terminal spikes. The flowers are nearly regular, open and the petals are connected towards the base. During the first year, it only produces a rosette of large leaves, six to fifteen inches long, similar to those of the Foxglove, but thicker and whitish with a soft, dense mass of hairs on both sides. In the following spring, a single, thick, pale stem, with tough, strong fibres enclosing a thin rod of white pith, grows out from the middle of the felted leaves. The leaves near the base of the stem are six to eight inches long and two to two and a half inches broad, and numerous, but become smaller further up the stem, where they grow on alternate sides. It is easy to identify the great mullein by the way the leaves hug the stem. The leaves are stalkless, broad and simple, with a wavy outline, their bases continuing down the stem, as in comfrey; the midrib from a quarter to half-way up the blade being actually joined to the stem. The leaf system is arranged in such a way that the smaller leaves above drop the rain onto the larger ones below, which direct the water to the roots. This is how the great mullein survives on dry soils. The hairs which cover the leaves so thickly are branched in star-like patterns and act as a protective coat, retaining moisture, and defending the plant from insect attacks and grazing animals; but this moisture does tend to encourage mould. The stem is also covered in hairs, as are the calyces and the outside of the petals so that the whole plant appears whitish or grey.

Towards the top of the stalk, the small, woolly leaves merge into the thick, densely crowded flower-spike, usually one foot long. The flowers open here and there on the spike, not in regular progression from the base, as in the Foxglove. The flowers are stalkless, forming an irregular cup, nearly one inch across, the five rounded sulphur-yellow petals joined at the base to form a very short tube, which is enclosed in a woolly calyx, deeply cut into five lobes. Three of the five stamens are shorter than the other two and have a large number of tiny white hairs on their filaments. These hairs are full of sap, which might be an additional attractant to insects. The anthers at the ends of the three short hairy stamens are one-celled – the two longer, smooth ones have larger anthers. All kinds of insects are attracted by this plant, the Honey Bee, Humble Bee, some of the smaller wild bees and different species of flies.

Habitat

Great mullein, grows all over Europe and in temperate Asia as far as the Himalayas. The early settlers took Mullein seeds with them to America, where it grew and spread and became a naturalised weed in the eastern States. It lives on hedge-banks, by roadsides and on waste ground, more especially on gravel, sand or chalk.

Season

It flowers during July and August.

How to Grow

It is easy to grow. Sow in ordinary soil and keep it free of weeds. Your only problem is likely to be slugs, which love it.

Parts Used

Leaves, flowers, root. Collect in July as it begins to flower. Dry the leaves and add them to boiling water for tea, then strain the tea through a fine cloth to remove the tiny hairs, which can irritate the throat.

Properties

Mullein is demulcent, emollient, astringent, slightly sedative, anti-spasmodic, narcotic, analgesic, anti-histaminic, anti-inflammatory, anti-cancer, antioxidant, anti-viral, anti-bacterial, oestrogenic, fungicide, hypnotic and sedative. The leaves, root, and the flowers are anodyne, antiseptic, diuretic, expectorant, nervine and vulnerary.

Chemical Constituents

Verbascum thapsus contains a cornucopia of valuable compounds which scientists from all over the world have been isolating and identifying for several decades. Both the leaves and flowers contain mucilage, which is soothing to irritated membranes. It contains many iridoid glycosides, including verbascoside, first isolated from the leaves in 1940 by Murakami, and aucubin, laterioside, harpagoside and ajugol. It contains a number of phenylethanoid glycosides, including forsythoside.

The flowers contain sterols, including beta sitosterol, according to Zhang in 1996.

There are many different types of terpenes in *V thapsus,* according to Hussainet in 2009, including sesquiterpenes and diterpenes. The plant contains several flavonoids, including luteolin, kaempferol, quercetin and rutin, which are antioxidant, according to Danchul in 2007. Mullein contains saponins, which are anti-microbial, anti-tumour and anti-viral. It contains carbohydrates and minerals.

Mullein seed oils contain high levels of gamma tocopherol (vitamin E) according to Parry in 2006 and high levels of polyunsaturated fatty acid, primarily linoleic acid. Polyunsaturated fatty acids are important components of cell walls; our cells need them for sending signals and expressing genes. Our cells also need polyunsaturated fatty acids in order to synthesise prostaglandins which are essential for a healthy nervous, endocrine, and immune system, according to Yehuda in 2001 and Parryet in 2006. In 1978 Pascual isolated palmitic, stearic, oleic, linoleic, linolenic, arachidic, and behenic acids and β-sitosterol from benzene extract of seed oil of *V. thapsus.* The plant also contains vitamin C and tannins.

Research

Scientists the world over have carried out research on *V thapsus,* almost all of it in the laboratory. Extracts of the plant protect cells from free radicals, according to Kumar and Singh in 2011 and Narayanaswamy and Balakrishnan, also in 2011. Extracts of the seed oil also protect cells from free radicals, according to Parry in 2006. In 1999 Ota and his team found that *V thapsus* extracts stopped sebum from oxidising, thus preventing body smell. In 2002 McCune and Johns found that root extract of *V thapsus* had anti-diabetes effect *in vitro*. All these experiments point to *V thapsus* being a rich source of antioxidants.

A number of different scientists have investigated the anti-bacterial power of *V thapsus* flowers and leaves, including Turker and Camper in 2002, Khan and his team in 2011, and Kumar and Singh in the same year, all of whom found that extracts of the plant were active against a number of different bacteria. Both Meurer-Grimes in 1996 and Speranza in 2010 agreed that the saponins in *V thapsus* were responsible for the anti-bacterial action of the extracts. In 2002 Sandra found that extracts of flowers and leaves of *V thapsus* were active against mycobacteria (the bacteria that cause tuberculosis). In 2011 Khan found that *V thapsus* was active against various fungi.

Several scientists, including Zanon in 2002, found that *V thapsus* extracts were powerfully anti-viral. Skwarek in 1979 found that the flowers had the most powerful effect. In 1995 McCutcheon demonstrated that plant extracts were anti-viral against herpes virus and in 2009 Rajbhandari found that extracts killed the influenza virus.

In 2002 Lin found *V thapsus* extracts stopped liver cancer cells from growing and multiplying. In 1988 Kawamo isolated a flavone from *V thapsus* which is anti-asthmatic, anti-allergic and anti-cancer. In 1999 Aboutabl found that polysaccharides extracted from *V thapsus* reduced cholesterol. In 2007 Ito found that extracts of the *V thapsus* leaves stimulated the hair outer root sheath to grow, so it should make a good hair tonic. A tincture of *V thapsus* dried leaves promotes healthy hair according to Roia in 1966. In 1997 Williams patented a skin treatment formula containing *V thapsus*. In 2001 Ohara patented a cosmetic bath preparation and detergent herbal formula containing *V thapsus*. Several Chinese scientists have investigated verbascoside, including Deng in 2008 who found that it protected nerve cells from damage, and Liao in 1999, who found that it helped muscles to resist fatigue. Li in 1999 found that verbascoside reduced oxidative stress in muscle caused by exhausting exercise, by decreasing the concentration of free radicals. Zho in 2012 found that verbascoside removed free radicals from heart muscle and protected the heart and skeletal muscle from free radical damage. Chen in 2002 found that iso-verbascoside stopped cancer cells from multiplying. It's difficult to say how much this was due to the mullein and how much to the various other ingredients in the formula he used. In 2012 Niaz and his team found that *V. thapsus* extracts killed roundworms (*Ascaridia galli*) and tapeworms (*Raillietina spiralis*) *in vitro*. In 2011 Mehdinezhad and his team found that *Verbascum thapsus* ointment had a good healing effect on rabbits' skin.

In 2001 and 2003 Sarrell and his team carried out two clinical trials, giving children suffering from earache either anaesthetic ear drops (amethocaine, phenazone and glycerine) or herbal extract ear drops (*Allium sativum, Verbascum thapsus, Calendula flores* and *Hypericum perforatum* in olive oil). They found that the herbal extract reduced the pain as much as the anaesthetic ear drops.

How to Use
Mullein is a powerful herb to strengthen the lungs and keep the bronchi healthy and free of infections. Take a mullein leaf infusion to treat sore throats, bronchitis, dry coughs and colds. To make a cough syrup, gently boil a cup of dried leaves in a cup of water until half of the water is gone. Strain through a cloth, pushing all the liquid out. Add 2 tablespoons of honey and mix well. Take 1 teaspoon every 3 or 4 hours.

Use mullein infusion for headaches, neuralgia and painful inflammatory conditions such as arthritis, rheumatism and gout because it encourages the kidneys to eliminate toxins and uric acid and it reduces inflammation in the joints. Take mullein tea to relieve tension, pain, anxiety and to relax and encourage restful sleep. Take mullein infusion for nervous palpitations, cramp and nervous colic. Its astringent properties are useful to treat nervous diarrhoea. Use mullein as a soothing diuretic, for burning and frequency of urination in cystitis and for fluid retention. But if cystitis persists, go to see a medical doctor.

Mullein oil is soothing and destroys bacteria, fungi and viruses. To make mullein flower oil, lay mullein flowers out to wilt, then crush them slightly and pack them into a jar. Fill the jar with olive or sunflower seed oil, submerging them completely and make sure there are no air bubbles. Cap the jar and place it on a sunny windowsill for at least five days, or up to a month. Then, strain the mixture and pour the oil into another jar. Mullein flower oil will keep for up to two years in a cool place. Use the oil infusion as earache drops, for catarrhal deafness and tinnitus, ear infections, wax accumulation and headache caused by congestion in the ears.

Make an ointment by melting wax together with the infused oil and use it to treat wounds and haemorrhoids. Its astringent properties will stop the bleeding and it will help to heal, soften and soothe irritated skin, shrink tissues, prevent secretion of fluids, enhance the elasticity and resistance of the skin, even restoring tissue in case of cell death.

Make a decoction of the roots to alleviate toothache, migraine headaches and relieve cramps and convulsions.

Dose

Mullein infusion: pour two pints of boiling water onto one ounce of dried mullein flowers and leaves, cover and leave to steep for four hours, or overnight. Then carefully strain through a cloth or a coffee filter to remove the hairs. Mullein infusion will last for 5-6 days refrigerated. To make it more palatable, mix it with a little peppermint and sweeten with honey. Take one teacupful three times a day.

Mullein extracts are available commercially in 250 mg/ml and

285 mg/ml dosages. Take up to 3 grams a day maximum dose.
Tincture: 20-30 drops three times a day.

Contraindications

Mullein is safe. But be careful to avoid the tiny hairs that cover
the entire plant by straining infusions and oils through muslin
or coffee filters. Traditionally people used mullein to treat
tuberculosis and kidney problems but anyone with tuberculosis
or kidney problems should see a medical doctor.

Chapter 9

Oak *Quercus robur*

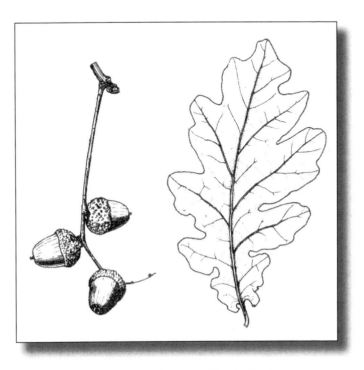

The old oak tree, battered and scarred by lightning from numerous thunderstorms, stood proudly overlooking the stream at the bottom of the Banky Meadow. When we were children we used to run down the hill to the stream where we played for hours on end, digging clay out of the bank to build dams like a tribe of little beavers, somehow dimly aware of its presence, although we paid very little attention to its crinkly bark and leafy branches. It was just part of the environment, had been for hundreds of years, sheltering myriads of insects, birds, animals, both small and large, holding the soil with its spreading roots, soaking up the rain, channelling it into the deep recesses of the earth.

I never knew how many hundreds of years old it was, but

it was a venerable tree with spreading branches wonderfully covered in leaves, which fell every autumn, to show its intricate skeleton against the white winter snow. Our carthorses used to stand under the oak tree when it rained and one by one were struck by lightning during storms. The oak tree lived on, shedding a branch here and there. A rabbit dug a hole among its roots and in the summer its branches filtered the hot sun, providing us with cool dappled shade.

I remember my father taking me down the lane to the oak forest at the bottom of the farm, telling me how one hundred years ago the drovers walked for miles behind their pigs, bringing them to forage in the woodlands. Despite the long walk the pigs grew fat scratching around in the forest eating acorns. Pig grazing rights in oak woods were known as pannage. At the time of the ancient Celts, Britain was covered by oak forest. Up until Elizabethan times, people used oak to build houses. Our old farmhouse was an Elizabethan half-timbered hall house. The intervening spaces were filled with bricks, mortar, lath and plaster, all of which provided numerous spaces for rats, mice and small birds to live. The house was cold and draughty, built four hundred years ago as a great hall with a fireplace in the middle and a hole in the roof to let the smoke out. During the intervening years many floors had been built, to divide the space into rooms and a great, winding chimney funnelled the smoke up and out of the hall. But the oak timbers remained strong and hard, hidden within the walls.

Oak trees grow all over Europe but the British adopted this tree as an emblem of Britishness, even engraving an oak twig on their sixpences one hundred years ago, when sixpences were made of silver and were worth something.

In ancient Britain oak trees were sacred to the Celts and their Druids and, according to Mrs Grieve, the name Quercus derives from the Celtic 'quer', meaning fine and 'cuez', meaning tree. According to Pliny the Druids cut mistletoe from the branches of the oak, dressed in ceremonial robes. But mistletoe, although it grows on many trees with softer wood, planted by birds as they wipe their beaks in the branches of the trees where they sit eating the berries, does not naturally grow in oak trees. This suggests that the wise Druids were cultivating it in their favourite tree, the sacred oak.

The Physicians of Myddvai said:

The oak will supply a variety of remedies, for all diseases proceeding from weakness in the nerves, spinal marrow and brain. Remedies are procured from the oak in a variety of ways.

Take fresh chips of oak, and macerate in running water, till their virtues be extracted; then take them out and put in some fresh chips, treating them as before. This being done nine times, boil the liquor to the half, put in a pound of honey to each two gallons and ferment. A quantity equal to the honey or any less quantity of a decoction of mistletoe, may be added if there is any at hand; but if not, it will be a very excellent drink nevertheless, and is called Oak Beer. It is the best drink of any to strengthen the body, constitution, nerves, brain and spinal marrow. It will also cure the diseases which proceed from weakness, a good draught being drank every morning fasting.

The inner bark of the oak is an excellent tonic... Take ripe acorns, let them be very crisply roasted, and kept in a well covered oak vessel. ... three table spoonfuls of this powder should be boiled in a good draught of goat's or kine's milk, then drank mixed with honey night and morning ... It is useful for uterine haemorrhage in women, for eruptions in all manner of men and for diseased lungs...

Gather the leaves of the oak in August or September, dry well, and keep covered. If applied to any contused integument, or watery excoriation, they will heal it. Take roasted acorns, or the inner bark roasted ground with bread corn, and make bread therewith. This bread is the best of any to strengthen a man's body, and to remove all complaints resulting from the winter cold or humidity.

This description by the Physicians of Myddvai suggests that the ancient Celts and their Druids used oak as a medicine, as well as revering it as one of their most sacred trees, represented by the letter Duir (D) in the Druid's Tree Alphabet. Susun Weed says that an oak wand is used magically to maintain a strong centre under adverse conditions, or to help to create openings to new realms of understanding.

Oak trees grow slowly but if they survive they can live up to two thousand years, spreading out their branches all around them. According to Mrs Grieve the trunk of the famous Fairlop Oak in Hainault Forest measured thirty-six feet, and her branches spread out over a circumference of three hundred feet. She said that the trunk of the Courthorpe Oak in Yorkshire measured seventy feet. King Arthur's Round Table was made from a single slice of oak, cut from an enormous bole, and is still shown at Winchester.

Botanical Description

Oak trees have pale green leaves with four or five lobes on each side and very short stalks. Acorns, on the other hand, have long stalks, called peduncles, which is why the common oak is also called the pedunculate oak. Large old oaks often have dead branches at the top because during years when there is a drought, they conserve water by not supplying their topmost branches and so manage to survive. The oak does not produce acorns until it has been growing for about fifty years. Then most of the acorns it does produce are eaten by animals. Only a few that forgetful squirrels have buried manage to grow.

Habitat

Oak trees grow wherever they can, often starting off life in a hedge in today's Britain, then being left to grow by the farmer, who subsequently removes the hedge, leaving the oak tree in the middle of a field. Their natural habitat is the forest, where they tower over smaller trees, shrubs and bushes.

Season

Oak trees clothe themselves in leaves sometime in the spring and shed them in the autumn.

How to Grow

You need to be very patient to grow oak trees and you need a large space for them to grow in. People used to plant oak trees for future generations to enjoy, since they grow so slowly, but few people have a large enough piece of land to contemplate growing oak trees.

Parts Used

The bark from the young twigs.

Preservation

Cut the bark from the young twigs, dry it away from the sun, then, when it is completely dry grind it up into a fine powder in a coffee grinder. You could extract the ground up bark into a mixture of alcohol and water 50/50, then either use it as a liquid extract or dry it out to make a dry extract. Or you can simply boil whole pieces of the dried bark to make a decoction.

Chemical Constituents

Oak bark contains anything between 8-20% tannins, depending on the time of the harvest, age of the branches and how they are extracted. Tannins are divided into: (i) galloyl esters and their derivatives (gallotannins, ellagitannins and complex tannins) and (ii) proanthocyanidins (condensed tannins). There are many different types of complex tannins and proanthocyanidins. Oak bark contains both types of tannins, according to many scientists, including Schofield in 2001. Different tannins have different effects: such as accelerating blood clotting, reducing harmful fats in the blood, lowering blood pressure and modulating immune responses. Proanthocyanidins are astringent because their polyhydroxy-phenolic groups cross-link with proteins.

Research

In 2010 the European Medicines Agency (EMA) assessed the bark of three oak species, including *Quercus robur,* because herbalists in several countries had been using it as a medicine for centuries. The EMA listed some of the laboratory research that scientists have been carrying out on oak bark. In 1986 Verhaeren and Lemli extracted gallotannins (now called hydrolysable tannins) from oak bark and demonstrated *in vitro* that these compounds had an astringent action on the proteins in the wall of the gut, forming a protective layer. In 2001 Carbonaro demonstrated *in vitro* that tannic acid (one of the tannins in oak bark) did not pass through the gut wall but bound to the proteins in the lining of the intestines. This protective layer of tannins prevents the gut from becoming inflamed and stops toxins from damaging the wall of the gut and escaping into the blood stream. In 1993 Pallenbach named proanthocyanidins as the type of tannin responsible for this effect. Several different scientists, including Khennouf in 2003, carried out *in vivo* tests which all proved that the bark of different oak species protected the wall of the gut. In 1999 in Jordan, Alkofahi and Atta demonstrated that the bark from various species of oak had an anti-ulcer effect *in vivo.* Several different scientists, including Yamasaki in 2007, demonstrated that tannins from oak were anti-viral *in vitro.*

Scientists have known for some time that tannins are anti-bacterial and anti-oxidant. Several scientists, including Rivas-Arreola and Rocha-Guzman in 2010 demonstrated *in vitro* that various oak bark tannins are anti-oxidant. Various scientists including Andrensek in 2004 and Mohan in 2008 have demonstrated that extracts of *Quercus robur* bark are anti-bacterial and anti-fungal.

Scientists, including Fridrich in 2008, demonstrated that oak tannins have a cancer preventative effect *in vivo*. This may be because carcinogens (cancer producing compounds) often produce free-radicals, which damage the cells in our bodies and many tannins scavenge these free radicals (get rid of them).

In 2014 Piwowarski and his team demonstrated that plants containing high levels of ellagitannins (including oak bark), caused the microbes in the gut to produce urolithins, anti-inflammatory compounds that can cross the gut wall and enter into the blood stream. Most of the tannins in oak bark, including ellagitannins, cannot pass through the gut wall but herbalists have been using oak bark to treat inflammatory diseases, such as rheumatism for centuries. Piwowarski's research may help explain how it can have an anti-inflammatory effect.

No one has yet carried out any clinical trials on oak bark, but the European Medicines Agency came to the conclusion that it is safe, especially at therapeutic doses and concentrations, if only used over short periods.

Properties

Oak bark preparations are astringent, local anaesthetic, anti-inflammatory and bring down fevers. When applied to burns and wounds, oak bark infusions form a protective layer which allows the damaged tissues to heal and since they are anti-bacterial and anti-fungal they will prevent wounds from becoming infected. They soothe gastritis and ulcers and cure mild diarrhoea. Gargling with an infusion of oak bark alleviates a sore throat.

How to Use

Take an infusion to treat diarrhoea, use as a mouth wash for minor inflammation or apply to the skin to soothe irritation. Use oak bark infusions to wash wounds and burns. Oak bark ointment is very effective for relieving the itching and burning of haemorrhoids. If you suffer from painful haemorrhoids you should always see a doctor before starting to use the oak bark ointment, just to make sure that you are not suffering from a serious condition.

Make a sitz bath with a quart of oak bark infusion to treat vaginitis: sore, inflamed vagina, which may be due to bacteria which cannot be detected, or too much sex. The oak bark will kill the bacteria, ease the pain and inflammation and tone the tissues. Use an oak bark sitz bath to ease haemorrhoids, fistulas and chronic pelvic pain.

Take half a cup of oak bark decoction three times a day to shrink goitre, reduce glandular inflammation, restore loss of voice and ease coughs, dry up mouth sores and bring down fever. Use oak bark decoction as a hair rinse to remove dandruff and encourage hair growth. Add oak bark decoction to your bath to heal varicose veins.

Make a poultice out of the young leaves to heal stings, bruises, ulcers, swellings and painful joints.

Dose

Boil four tablespoons of bark in two litres of water for ten minutes for a decoction.

Steep 5 grams in a litre of water for an infusion.

Tincture 1-2 ml three times a day.

Contraindications

A few people are allergic to oak bark and oak pollen. Do not use oak bark during pregnancy and lactation. Provided it is not used over long periods and only in the recommended dosage, oak bark is safe. If taken together with other herbs it may interfere with the uptake of alkaloids and it might inhibit iron absorption.

Chapter 10

Raspberry *Rubus idaeus*

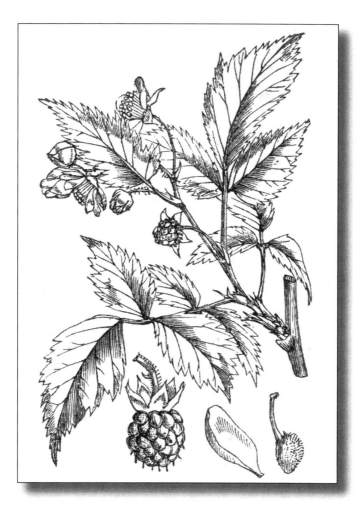

I've been growing raspberries in my garden for several years, on a fine south facing slope. I water them every day in the dry summer months and they reward me with wonderful quantities of fruit. There is something particularly British about raspberries, which enjoy our cool, wet climate and have been growing in

Britain since the Mesolithic Age, possibly longer. The Physicians of Myddvai used the leaves and the fruit as medicine and I can imagine the ancient Celts foraging for raspberries and blueberries in the forests.

Botanical Description

Raspberries are another member of the Rosaceae, which also includes blackberries. The perennial root stock sends up biennial stems, which produce leaves in the first year and flowering side shoots and five-petalled white flowers in the summer of the second year. They spread out their roots sideways and send up secondary shoots, quickly colonising large areas of ground up to ten metres square. The stems are straight with prickles all along them, though when they grow tall, they start to bend over. The leaves have three to seven oval, pointed leaflets, which are white and softly hairy on the underside, smooth and green on the upper side. The fruit is a collection of little red drupelets, each containing a seed. Both the leaves and the fruit are medicinal.

Habitat

Wild raspberries grow all over Britain, including Scotland, in thickets, clearings and open woods.

Season

Harvest the leaves in June, before the fruit ripens. Wild raspberries are ready to pick in July and August.

How to Grow

Plant bare rooted plants about thirty centimetres deep in well dug and manured soil, preferably in a sunny place. There are summer fruiting and autumn fruiting varieties, both of which need to be pruned back after the harvest is finished. In our windy British climate they do need to be supported by strong posts three metres apart, with galvanised wire stretched across the posts to hold up the canes. Since the roots spread underground you will have to keep digging up rogue raspberry canes that will sprout out through the lawn, flower bed or anywhere else that they can go!

Parts Used
Leaves and fruit.

Preservation
Pick the leaves and lay them out to dry on racks away from the sun.

Properties
Raspberry leaf is astringent and antibacterial and can be used internally and externally. It is tonic to a sluggish digestive system and atonic bowel in children. Infusion of Raspberry Leaf can help alleviate the symptoms of gingivitis or gum disease. Many women claim that it helps ease the symptoms of PMS and herbalists believe that astringent herbs strengthen the tissues, especially the tissues of the uterus. This is why they recommend raspberry leaf during the last few weeks of pregnancy to prepare a woman for giving birth.

Chemical Constituents of the Leaves
The leaves contain 4.6% tannins, including ellagic acid, sanguiin H6, lambertianin C, Lambertianin D, according to Patel in 2004 and 0.44% flavonoids, including quercetin glycosides, mainly hyperoside and kaempferol glycosides, according to Gudej and Tomczyk in the same year. The leaves also contain magnesium, potassium, iron and B-vitamins, pectin, citric and malic acid, and the mysterious 'fragarine'.

Chemical Constituents of the Fruit
The fruit contains ellagitannins, such as sanguiin H6 and lam-

bertianin according to Beekwilder; flavonoids and anthocyanins, according to Anttonen and Karjalainen in 2005 and Mazu in 2014. They also contain vitamins A, B, C, E, sugars, iron, calcium, phosphorus and volatile compounds including α-pinene, camphene, β-myrcene and limonene.

Raspberry Fruit Research

Anthocyanins give raspberries their colour and are antioxidant. They also contain antioxidant vitamin C. In 2000 Wang and Lin found that as the fruit ripened they had more and more anthocyanins in them and they became more and more antioxidant. They found that young raspberry leaves were more than twice as powerfully antioxidant as the raspberry fruit but as the leaves aged, they lost their antioxidant properties. Antioxidants counteract oxidative stress, which is caused by free radicals. We are constantly exposed to free radicals from air pollution, food additives, pesticides, radiation and a number of other modern day toxins. Oxidative stress can damage our cells and may contribute towards the development of all sorts of diseases, including cancer, cardiovascular diseases, Alzheimer's disease, Parkinson's disease and eye diseases such as cataracts and age-related macular degeneration. In 2002 Liu and his team compared four varieties of raspberries and found that the Heritage variety was the reddest and had the highest amounts of phenolic compounds, the most flavonoids and the most anthocyanins. This variety was the most antioxidant and inhibited human liver cancer cells from dividing and multiplying.

Ellagitannins in ripe raspberries are also antioxidant, as well as antibacterial, according to Puupponen-Pimia in Finland in 2005. In 2001 Ryan and his team found that a 1:5 dilution of raspberry juice and raspberry juice cordial inhibited eleven bacteria, including *Salmonella enteritidis, in vitro.*

Raspberry Leaf Research

There has been very little research on raspberry leaf, apart from a few laboratory studies such as the one carried out in 1970 by Bamford, who found that raspberry leaf extract stimulated contractions in human uterine tissue. For twenty minutes the contractions became normal but less frequent and more regular. But the hormone oxytocin stimulates contractions during labour so this study may have no relevance to labour. In 2009 Johnson gave an oral dose of raspberry leaf (10mg/kg per day), quercetin, kaempferol or control to 40 Wistar rats. This made no differences to the survival or weight of the rat babies when they were born but the pregnancies lasted longer. He also found that the females in the next generation of offspring had a significantly earlier puberty. But it was a very small trial, involving only 20 rats, rats are completely different from humans, and they were given the raspberry leaf from conception, rather than during the last weeks of pregnancy, so it is difficult to see whether the results of this study have any relevance.

More interesting than this rat research was the survey carried out in 1999 by McFarlin of 500 nurse-midwives in the USA. He found that, of the ninety who replied, sixty-three per cent had given their patients red raspberry leaf to stimulate labour, particularly in home births or birth centres. Sixty-nine per cent of the midwives had learned about the use of raspberry from colleagues but only twenty-two per cent recorded that they had used herbs. In 2006 Forster carried out a survey of five hundred and eighty-eight women who visited an antenatal clinic in Melbourne, Australia at around thirty-seven weeks. He found that thirty-six per cent of the women were taking a herbal supplement and fourteen per cent were taking raspberry leaf.

In the same year Parsons compared fifty-seven women who had taken raspberry leaf tea (or tablets) with fifty-one women from the same hospital who had not, and found that the babies from both groups were fine. But the women who took the raspberry leaf tea tended to give birth without forceps or emergency caesarians more often than the women who hadn't taken the raspberry leaf. Since this study looked promising, in 2001 Simpson carried out a double-blind, randomised, placebo controlled trial in a hospital in Sydney, Australia. Two hundred and forty low-risk women who were expecting their first baby began the trial and 192 completed it. They took raspberry leaf tablets (1.2g/day) or placebo from 32 weeks until birth. The women who took the raspberry leaf tablets had a shorter second stage of labour and fewer forceps deliveries but the number of women who took part in the study was too small to convince the scientific world that raspberry leaf is helpful to women giving birth.

How to Use

I'm sure I don't need to encourage you to eat raspberries, but since they are so expensive, why not grow them if you have a garden or an allotment and if you live in a nice cool climate such as Britain. If you grow the early and the late varieties you can enjoy their delicious fruit from July until October. The fruits are a valuable food with antibacterial and anti-oxidant properties.

Use the leaves to treat children for mild diarrhoea, use as a mouth wash for oral thrush, mouth ulcers and gum infections. Many midwives and herbalists continue to recommend raspberry leaf tea during the last three months of pregnancy to prepare the womb for birth, but the scientific world remains sceptical as to whether this actually has any effect. However, Susun Weed says that raspberry leaf tea tones the uterus and helps to prevent haemorrhage after the birth. She says that it tones the muscles used during labour and encourages the uterus to let go, so that the delivery is quicker. It does not strengthen contractions, but does allow the contracting uterus to work more effectively and so may make the birth easier and faster.

Dose

4-8g dried leaf three times a day.

Infusion of raspberry leaves: 2 teaspoons of dried herb in one cup of boiling water, left to steep 10-15 minutes. 3-4 pints a week in the last 3 months and a full pint of hot tea when labour begins.

Contraindications

Raspberries and raspberry leaves are safe and non toxic.

Chapter 11

Red clover *Trifolium pratense*

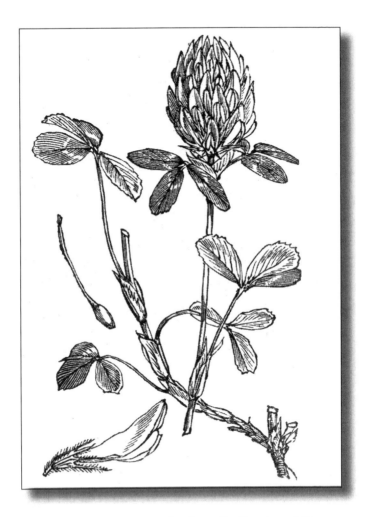

Red clover is an ancient British plant. In Greek and Roman my-
thology the three-leaf clover represents the triad goddesses and
in mediaeval times the four leafed clover symbolised complete
happiness, according to Onstad. Each leaf represents a different aspect of happiness: fame, wealth, faithful lover and good

health. Red clover used to be a common sight in pastures all over Britain but since farmers have been sowing wild white clover with their grasses it has become less common.

Botanical Description
It's a member of the Leguminosae, the nitrogen fixing bean family. Each red clover plant has several stems one to two feet high, slightly hairy with the characteristic three leafletted leaves. The flowers are red to purple, fragrant, short-stalked or stalkless, round or ovoid and about 10-15 mm long. The flowers have lots of little bell-shaped calyces very close together with five linear lobes; the petals are about twice the calyx length.

Habitat
Red clover is a short lived perennial plant that tends to grow in old meadows that have been left to flourish with an abundance of different species of plants, including many different grasses. You can still find it in wild places, grass verges and uncultivated places in Britain. Settlers from Britain brought it to North America where it has spread and made its home.

Season
Wild red clover flowers between May and the end of summer, but if you grow it you can crop it three times a year.

How to Grow
Red clover prefers well drained, damp, slightly acidic soil. It doesn't like a lot of manure or artificial fertiliser or being over grazed. Bumble bees like it. It grows best in a mixture of grasses and you can sow it any time of the year.

Parts Used
The flower heads.

Preservation

Pick the flower heads and dry them in a warm, airy place away from the sun. You can make a tincture using 45% alcohol and 55% water. Some types of vodka contain 45% alcohol.

Properties

Red clover is a skin alterative and sedative, according to *Potter's New Cyclopedia of Drugs and Preparations*. It restores normal function to the liver, kidneys, lungs and digestive tract, so that they are better able to eliminate toxins. This restores the skin to a radiant, healthy condition. It also restores the nervous system, thus relaxing both body and mind. Red clover is rich in phyto-oestrogens and herbalists believe that it helps minimise menstrual cramps by bringing the body's hormone levels into better balance. It can relieve hot flushes, prevent osteoporosis and alleviate ovarian cysts, possibly even improve libido in some menopausal women.

Chemical Constituents

Red clover contains 0.17% isoflavones, which are phyto-oestrogens (water-soluble chemicals that act like oestrogens): formonetin, biochanin A, daidzein, genistein, coumestrol, naringen, pratensein, trifoside, irilone, isoquercitrin, calycosine galactoside and pectolinarin, according to Lin in 2000. Formonetin and biochanin are precursors of genistein and daidzein. Biochanin A has anti-tumour properties, according to John M. Cassady.

It also contains coumarins, carbohydrates, flavonoids (isohamnetin, kaempferol, quercetin and their glycosides), saponins: soya-sapogenols B-F, Vitamins A, C, B-complex and minerals: calcium, chromium, iron and magnesium.

Research

Doctors frequently prescribe Hormone Replacement Therapy (HRT) to allay the symptoms of menopause such as hot flushes, night sweats, insomnia and cognitive dysfunction, as well as to protect against bone loss and ischemic heart disease, caused by falling oestrogen levels. But HRT can cause breast or uterine cancer, heart attacks, coronary attacks and strokes. Asian women, who eat soya products on a regular basis are less likely to suffer from breast cancer, osteoporosis, heart disease and stroke than women in the West. Scientists believe that this is due to the isoflavones, or plant oestrogens, present in the soya products that they eat, since there is evidence that isoflavones alleviate menopausal symptoms. Most of the scientific research has focussed on soya beans but all the members of the bean family, the Leguminosae, including red clover, contain isoflavones. So scientists began to investigate the chemical constituents of red clover, which contains a number of different isoflavones that also produce oestrogen-like effects. Like soya, red clover does not produce the same side effects as HRT. Scientists were only interested in the oestrogen-like qualities of the isoflavones in red clover, not in the whole flower with all its other healing properties. So all the research was based on standardising certain isoflavones in red clover extract and testing the extract on men and women suffering from various different symptoms. In 2003 Huntley and Ernst reviewed the literature and came to the conclusion that red clover may help certain menopausal symptoms.

In 2002 Van de Weijer and Barentsen carried out a double blind clinical trial on 30 post-menopausal women who were experiencing more than five hot flushes per day. They found that a red clover extract reduced the frequency and severity of hot flushes by about fifty per cent compared to placebo. This was a small but well designed trial which showed that 12 weeks of 80 mg per day of Promensil (Novogen) (an extract of red clover containing very accurately determined amounts of the principal isoflavanoids: biochanin A, formononetin, genistein and daidzein (total isoflavanoid content of 40 mg per tablet)) did not have any adverse effects. Jeri in the same year also carried out a double blind clinical trial and achieved the same results. In 2001 Clifton-Bligh and his team gave various doses of Rimostil, to forty-six post menopausal women. Rimostil contained the isoflavones: genistein, daidzein, formononetin, and biochanin. After six months they found that the women who took the higher doses of Rimostil had more high density lipoprotein (good fats) in their blood and their two lower arm bones were denser and stronger. In 2004 Atkinson and her team carried out a double blind clinical trial with two hundred and five post-menopausal women, giving them Promensil for one year. The study demonstrated that, at this low dose of Promensil, breast density did not increase in women who already had increased breast density. This was encouraging since HRT does increase breast density, which can lead to breast cancer. One hundred and seventy-seven women finished the trial and those taking the red clover isoflavones lost less bone than the women taking the placebo. The isoflavones might have even helped build bone in these post-menopausal women.

In 2003 Howes and his team gave 50 mg/day of isoflavones from red clover to sixteen postmenopausal women with type two diabetes for four weeks compared to placebo. The women taking the red clover isoflavones had lower blood pressure than the women taking the placebo. Also in 2003 Teede and her team carried out a randomised, double-blind trial, giving isoflavones to eighty healthy subjects for two six-week periods. As people age, in many cases, the walls of their arteries become stiffer and less flexible due to the buildup of fatty plaques and atheroschlerosis. This can lead to high blood pressure. Teede found that the artery walls of the people taking the isoflavones were less stiff and more elastic and their pulse rates were slower than those of the people taking the placebo. These isoflavones did not affect blood pressure. In 2002 Ingram and his team carried out a double blind trial, giving isoflavones to women who were suffering from breast pain before and during their periods. Nine out of the twelve women taking the isoflavones said that their breast pain was less severe. Interestingly although isoflavones have an oestrogenic effect in post-menopausal women, they have a weak anti-oestrogen effect in pre-menopausal women.

About fifty per cent of men over fifty suffer from enlarged prostate or prostate cancer, the second most common cause of death from cancer in the United States. In 1998 Griffiths suggested that there was epidemiological evidence that the diet enjoyed by Asian men from China, Japan and Thailand, which is rich in isoflavones, protects them from prostate cancer.

In 2016 Jarred and his team gave 160 mg/day isoflavones from red clover to thirty-eight men with prostate cancer. After the prostates had been removed they found that there were more dead tumour cells in the prostates of the men who had taken the isoflavones than in those of the men who had not. So isoflavones in the diet may prevent prostate cancer from progressing by causing the body to kill the cancer cells in low to moderate-grade tumours. This might be one of the reasons why fewer Asian men tend to suffer from prostate cancer. There were no side effects.

Tumours need a blood supply in order to grow so they send out biochemical signals that coax the body into growing blood vessels right into them, a process called angiogenesis. According to James Duke, the American ethnobotanist, Genistein, one of the isoflavones from red clover, seems to interfere with this process.

In 2001 Widyarini and his team suggested that red clover or *Trifolium pratense* could be used as an acne remedy because of its anti-inflammatory flavonoids.

How to Use

Make an infusion of red clover flowers to calm your nerves before menstruation and relieve menstrual cramps and breast pain during menstruation. It is particularly good for relieving the symptoms of menopause, such as hot flushes, mood changes and nervous irritability and quite safe to drink on a regular basis, as long as you do not exceed the dosage. It will also protect your bones from osteoporosis and your blood vessels from accumulating fatty plaques. Infusions of the flowers will help purify the blood and prevent teenage skin from breaking out in spots. Add red clover flowers to the infusions you make to help you get over coughs and colds. Make it into ointments to treat psoriasis, eczema and rashes and to accelerate wound healing.

Dose

Make an infusion of red clover using half an ounce to an ounce of red clover to two pints of boiling water, cover and allow to steep overnight.

40-80 mg/day of extract with standardised isoflavones: biochanin A, formononetin, genistein and daidzein.

Contraindications

Do not use if you have had breast cancer, if you are pregnant or breastfeeding or if you are taking oral contraceptives, oestrogen, or progesterone therapies. According to James Duke, this herb's oestrogens are so concentrated that women should take care with the dosage. People who have overdosed on isoflavones have suffered swelling of the ankles and feet, abdominal tenderness and loss of appetite.

Chapter 12

Dog rose *Rosa canina*

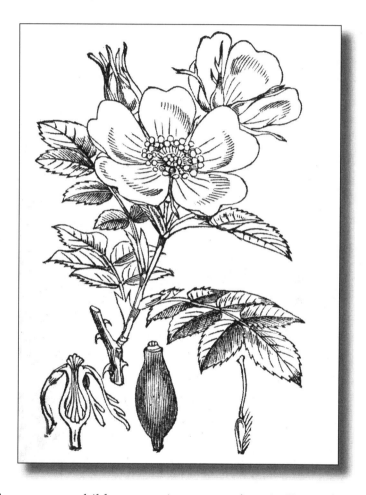

When we were children, growing up on a farm in Kent, we used to go out on winter's days to look for ripe rose hips. I remember how excited we were to find the first soft rose hips which we could pick to squeeze out the sticky fruit pulp into our mouths, carefully leaving the hairy pips behind.

The dog rose has been growing in Britain since before the last

Ice Age. Hundreds of years ago European colonisers brought it to America, where it escaped cultivation, naturalised and now grows wild. The Physicians of Myddvai used rose water, which suggests that the ancient Celts also made use of it.

Flower of perfection, symbol of love, famed in many mythologies, highly prized by poets, the rose was dedicated to the Goddess of love and war: Ishtar in Babylonia, Isis in Egypt, Aphrodite in Greece and Venus in Rome. Ancient Muslim tradition says that the rose comes from the sweat and tears of the prophet Mohammed. As Aphrodite, the goddess of love emerged from the sea, roses grew from the foam. When she ran to save her lover, Adonis, from a wild boar sent by jealous Ares to kill him, she became entangled in thorn bushes in her haste and roses grew from her spilt blood. Dante designed paradise, in his Divine Comedy, in the shape of a rose. In the ninth-century Zoroastrian scripture Bundahishn (Original Creation), each listed plant was associated with a particular angel. Dog rose belonged to the Zoroastrian angel of justice, who judged the souls of the dead.

Mrs Grieve tells the story of the wedding feast of the son of Akbar, the Mughal Emperor in sixteenth-century India. Akbar ordered his servants to dig a canal around the wedding garden and to fill it with rose water. In the hot sun the oil separated from the water and its exquisite perfume was realised, captured and shortly afterwards manufactured. I cannot imagine how they could have captured the rose oil from a moat! Another fantastical story relates how the Druids anointed the sacred stones of Stone Henge with rose oil. The process of distillation had not yet been invented at the time of the Druids.

Rosa canina is the second most frequently mentioned medicinal plant in the Chilandar Medical Codex, the significant medieval Serbian pharmacological manuscript on European medical science from the twelfth to the fifteenth centuries.

Botanical Description

The dog rose is a member of the Rosaceae, a family that includes the apple, cherry, plum, strawberry, raspberry and many of the other delightful British summer fruits. It grows as a large shrub or small tree with arching stems, up to nine feet (2.74 metres). It has prickly stems with pinnate, deciduous leaves with stipules. Pink or white flowers with five petals grow out of the ends of the stems. Dog roses have strong roots that spread underground and they are very hardy. In autumn they produce rose hips: red, oval, pointed receptacles swollen to form the flesh of the hip, which does not fuse with the hairy pips inside. It is the opposite of the strawberry, in which the receptacle swells to form a cushion, pushing the seeds to the outside.

Habitat

Dog roses grow in hedges and on the edges of woodland in Britain.

Season

Dog rose flowers in June and July. The fruit appears in September and October but doesn't ripen until later in the year.

How to Grow

If you want to grow dog roses from seed you need to be patient since they will take a couple of years to germinate. Broadcast the seed quite densely: aim for about two centimetres between seeds. Firm with a roller or board to press the seed well into the soil. Cover with five millimetres of grit and keep the seeds moist. Once the seeds start to germinate they will grow quickly, as long as they are watered regularly. Dog rose will grow in chalky, sandy, clay or loamy soil, at almost any pH, as long as it is moist and well drained and makes a good addition to a hedge. In parts of North America there are regulations against growing it, due to the way it spreads so uncontrollably.

Parts Used

The flowers and the rose hips.

Preservation

Dry the rose petals and the rose hips. As soon as the rose petals are dry store them in a glass container out of the light. The rose hips will take longer to dry.

Properties

Rose petals lift the spirits with their perfume. They are mildly astringent and antioxidant, so can be used to strengthen a weak stomach and for diarrhoea, for sore mouth and throat.

Rose hips are a valuable source of vitamin C in the winter. They are astringent, antibacterial, anti-inflammatory, antioxidant and used for colds, diabetes, diarrhoea, oedema, fever, gastritis, gout, rheumatism, sciatica. Rose hip powder, taken regularly will cure rheumatoid arthritis, prevent atheroschlerosis and lessen the pain of osteoarthritis.

Chemical Constituents

Petals

Roses contain small amounts of volatile oils: in 2007 in Iran, Tabaei-Aghdaei found between 0.017-0.35% in damask roses. The British dog rose contains even smaller amounts. These volatile oils are complex, containing at least ninety-five different compounds, and in 2008 Jalali-Heravi identified a few of these: citronellol, nerol, geraniol, linalool.

In 1991 Velioglu and Mazza found 2.85% anthocyanins.

In 2006 Vinokur found about 8% gallic acid in rose teas.

In 2008 Kumar identified the flavonoids: rutin, quercitrin, myricetin, kaempferol.

Hips

Rose hips contain the anti-inflammatory galactolipid: (2S)-1,2-

di-O-[(9Z,12Z,15Z)-octadeca-9,12,15-trienoyl]-3-O- β-D-galacto-
pyranosyl glycerol (GOPO), vitamin C, A, B3, D, E, phenolic
compounds, and carotenoids such as: lycopene, lutein, zeaxan-
thin; amino acids, flavonoids, pectins, sugars, tannins, tocopherol, beta sitosterol and long-chain polyunsaturated fatty acids,
magnesium and copper. The flavonoids and organic acids keep
the vitamin C stable by inhibiting oxidation.

One hundred grams of Hyben Vital rose hip powder from
Denmark contains five hundred milligrams of vitamin C, 5.8g
pectin, 5.8mg beta-crotene, 50 mg beta-sitosterol, 0.2 mg folic
acid, 4.6 mg vitamin E, 170 mg magnesium, 1 mg zinc and 10.9
ug copper.

Preservation

Collect the petals in early summer and spread them out to dry.
Pick the hips in late autumn, early winter, when they are soft
and ripe. Dry them in a warm, airy place away from the sun.

Research

Scientists have carried out masses of research on rose hip
powder, mostly looking at its anti-rheumatic properties, since it
contains powerful anti-inflammatory compounds.

At least nine double-blind, placebo-controlled clinical studies have investigated how effective Hyben Vital or Litozin rose
hip powder is for treating osteoarthritis, high cholesterol levels, Crohn's disease, chronic back and musculoskeletal pain, and
reducing C-reactive protein levels, which rise in the blood in
response to inflammation. Trials carried out in 2003, 2004 and
2005 showed that *R canina* hip powder reduces pain in osteoarthritis patients. A clinical trial carried out in 2006 demonstrated
that LitoZin reduced pain and inflammation in rheumatoid arthritis patients. Inflammation causes both pain and damage to
the joints, so reducing inflammation is essential for controlling
the disease. Another clinical trial carried out in 2013 by Winther

demonstrated that patients with osteoarthritis in their hands felt less pain and stiffness after taking rose hip powder. Patients with rheumatoid arthritis can definitely benefit from taking rose hip powder. Scientists need to carry out larger scale clinical trials to confirm these results.

From 2011 onwards pharmaceutical companies have been producing Litozin from seedless Chilean rose hips, with added vitamin C, carotenes, flavonoids, triterpenic acid and galacto-lipids (trade name Rosenoids). Scientists have only studied its effect on osteoarthritis.

In 2012 Andersson and his team observed that the blood pressure of patients taking rose hip powder during yet another osteoarthritis clinical trial went down. Their cholesterol levels were also lower after six weeks taking the rose hip powder. In 2001 Rein and his team found that patients who took rose hip powder in a clinical trial to treat osteoarthritis had less cholesterol in their blood.

In 1998 Stevensen used rose oil to treat acne and in 2010 Tsai and his team found that *Rosa damascene*, inhibited *P. acnes,* the bacterium which causes acne in teenagers. So adding rose oil to cosmetic products does more than merely adding a pleasant fragrance. It may well help to keep the skin clear of spots and pustules. In 2015 Phetcharat gave three grams of the rose hip powder mixed with yogurt to half the thirty-four women and placebo to the other half. After eight weeks, the skin of the group who had eaten the rose hip powder was less deeply lined, more elastic and moist. The scientists thought that the antioxidants in the rose hip powder may help maintain cell membranes, thus keeping cells alive.

How to Use

Use a tincture of roses for sore mouth and throat and as a calming digestive astringent.

Pick rose hips and make them into jams, jellies and syrups.

Dry them to use in teas and infusions.

Drink rose hip tea daily to benefit your skin, since rose hips contain plenty of vitamin A, which helps to regenerate skin cells, to heal wounds and scars and to keep the skin elastic and nourished. This will not only prevent wrinkles, but can actually help to minimise any that have already appeared.

Take rose hip powder or capsules to help prevent colds and coughs and help the immune system to fight off infections. Take rose hip as a daily supplement to keep your blood vessels clear from plaque, prevent rheumatoid arthritis, ease the pain of osteoarthritis and prevent the joints from degenerating further.

Dose

Tincture of roses 1:1 distilled and macerated as a cordial 5-10 ml per week.

Syrup of roses 30-100 ml.

Rose hips infusion: 100 g fresh or 45g dry.

Rose hip powder 5-10 g per day.

Contraindications

Rose hips are safe if taken in moderate doses. There have been cases of people who took forty grams a day of rose hip powder, who suffered some gastrointestinal disturbances. But this is way above the recommended dose!

Chapter 13

Shepherd's purse *Capsella bursa pastoris*

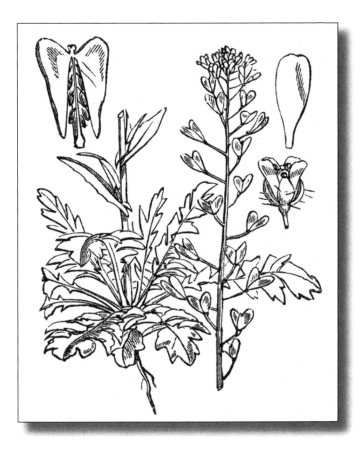

Shepherd's purse is another of those plants that has been growing in Britain for thousands of years. Tollund man (500 BCE-400
BCE) had shepherd's purse seeds in his stomach, according to
Bown, 1995. People have been eating it for at least eight thousand
years. Archaeobotanists found shepherd's purse seeds during an
excavation of the Catal Huyuk site in Turkey (5950 BCE). Its seed
pods look like old-fashioned leather purses. According to Mrs
Grieve the Irish called it 'Clappendepouch' since it looked like

the bell or clapper that lepers used when they stood at cross-roads, receiving their alms in a cup at the end of a long pole. The Pilgrim Fathers took the seed with them when they travelled to America. They planted it, it went to seed and spread and became naturalised.

Mrs Grieve says that shepherd's purse is one of the most important medicinal plants of the Cruciferae. She recommends an infusion of the dried leaves to stop haemorrhages of all kinds, in the stomach, the lungs or the uterus and especially bleeding from the kidneys. The Chinese and Japanese used it for many centuries, to stem the flow of blood, as a diuretic and to bring down a fever, according to Kuroda and Takagi in 1968. People used the whole plant to treat oedema caused by inflammation of the kidneys, pain while urinating, blood in the faeces, heavy bleeding at menstruation, chyluria (fat globules in the urine) and hypertension, according to Song in 2007. In some countries people eat the leaves and roots as a vegetable, raw or cooked, according to Kweon in 1996. Traditionally people have used a tea made from the whole plant to cure scurvy, to bring down blood pressure, as an astringent, diuretic, stimulant, to stop bleeding and to heal wounds. In China scientists have ranked it seventh out of two hundred and fifty potential anti-fertility plants. According to Schultz in 1998 the compound responsible for stemming the flow of blood seems to be an unspecified peptide.

Botanical Description

The main leaves are two to six inches long and either irregularly pinnatifid (composed of lots of little pointed leaflets) or entire with toothed edges. Before it flowers the leaves grow out from the centre of the plant, the outer ones flat on the ground, forming a rosette. When it flowers, a slender stem with a few branches, grows out of the centre of the leaves. The stem is smooth, except at the lower part, with a few, small, oblong leaves, arrow-shaped at the base, and above them numerous small, white, inconspicuous flowers, which are self-fertilised and followed by wedge-shaped fruit pods, divided by narrow partitions into two cells, which contain several oblong yellow seeds. When the seeds are ripe the pod splits open into two boat-shaped valves.

Habitat
It will grow in the poorest soil, remaining very small, but in good soil it will grow to two feet and flourishes in hedgerows, roadsides and waste ground.

Season
Most of the year, after the winter frosts have gone.

How to Grow
If you do want to grow it, sow the seeds in well dug, fertile soil, between February and May. Harvest the aerial part of the plant after a month, well before it flowers. Be careful not to let it go to seed or you will find it sowing itself everywhere.

Parts Used
The whole plant above ground.

Preservation
The fresh leaves are the best but you can dry the leaves, or make a tincture using twenty per cent alcohol to eighty per cent water.

Properties
Shepherd's purse is astringent, antioxidant, antibacterial, antifungal, anti-inflammatory and anti-ulcer.

Chemical Constituents
Shepherd's purse contains flavonoids, including luteolin and quercetin; glucosinolates, e.g., sinigrin; polypeptides, choline, acetylcholine, histamine and tyramine, according to Khare in

2007. It also contains proteins, linoleic acid and polyunsaturated fatty acid according to Zennie TM and Ogzewalla D.

James Duke found that 100g of the leaves contained 280 calories, 35.6 g protein, 4.2 g fat, 44.1 g carbohydrate; 10.2 g fibre, 21,949 mg vitamin A, 2.12 mg thiamine (B1), 1.44 mg riboflavin (B2), 3.4 mg niacin, and 305 mg vitamin C. He also found the following minerals and trace elements in one kilogram of the edible part of the plant: 0.70mg copper, 6.32 mg lead, 5.48 mg zinc 4.50 mg manganese, 0.15 mg cobalt, 224.4 potassium, 44.36 mg iron, 2.396 mg calcium and 2.90 mg sodium.

It also contains the isothiocyanate compound, sulforaphane, hemostyptic peptide and 0.02 per cent volatile oil.

Research

Scientists from many different countries have been researching the properties of shepherd's purse for several decades, but almost all of this research was carried out in laboratories. Many different teams have investigated its antibiotic properties, including those of El-Abyad in 1990, Park in 2000, Grosso in 2011, Alizadeh in 2012, Hasan 2013. Soleimanpour in 2013 and Choi in 2014, all of whom demonstrated that shepherd's purse extracts were antibacterial and antifungal.

Various scientists have investigated the anti-cancer properties of fumaric acid from shepherd's purse, including Kuroda and Akao in 1981, Kuroda in 1990, Khare in 2007, Yildirim, Karakas and Turker in 2012 and Lee in 2013, all of whom found that *C. bursa-pastoris* extracts inhibited tumours *in vitro*.

Since shepherd's purse is rich in flavonoids, we would expect it to be antioxidant, so it is no surprise that in 2011 Grosso demonstrated that *Capsella bursa-pastoris* extracts were efficient free radical scavengers and in 2013 Kubínova and his team demonstrated that extracts of shepherd's purse were antioxidant *in vitro*. In 1968 Kuroda and Takagi demonstrated that extracts of *Capsella bursa-pastoris* were anti-inflammatory and anti-ulcer *in vivo* and stimulated rat uterus like oxytocin. In 1971 Jurisson demonstrated that the plant stimulated guinea-pig small intestine. In 1981 Shipochliev demonstrated that water extracts of *Capsella bursa-pastoris* had a tonic effect.

In 1969 Kuroda and Takagi demonstrated that shepherd's purse increased blood flow to the coronary artery in dogs, slowed down the heart and weakened heart muscular contraction *in vitro*. In 2007 Khare isolated hesperidin and rutin from the young leaves. He demonstrated that these compounds reduced permeability of blood vessel walls.

In 2011 Ghoreschi and his team demonstrated that fumarates (compounds found abundantly in shepherd's purse) improve psoriasis and multiple sclerosis in mice. In 2007 Al Qasoumi demonstrated that *Capsella bursa-pastoris* protected the livers of rats. In 1971 Jurisson demonstrated that the plant had a sedative effect on mice. In 1955 East demonstrated that dried *Capsella bursa-pastoris,* made male and female mice infertile.

Unfortunately no one has carried out clinical trials using the whole shepherd's purse plant, although the laboratory results have amply demonstrated that it has numerous useful medicinal properties. Scientists have tended to focus on fumaric acid, isolated from the plant, and in 1989 Nieboer and his team investigated it for the treatment of psoriasis. They gave a fumaric acid compound to 36 patients suffering from psoriasis and said that it was rather effective. So they carried out several double blind studies with two fumaric acid compounds (monoethyl-fumaric acid ester sodium and dimethyl-fumaric acid ester.) They found that 720 mg monoethylfumaric acid ester reduced the scaling and itching but did not stop the eruption from spreading. 240 mg of dimethylfumaric acid ester, on the other hand, was more effective. Isolating an active compound from a plant may be of interest to the pharmaceutical companies, who hope to make profit from selling it, but the fumaric acid treatment had serious side effects: nausea, diarrhoea, general malaise, severe stomach ache, mild disturbances of liver and kidney function. Fifty per cent of the patients treated with dimethylfumaric acid ester suffered from abnormally low levels of white blood cells, especially suppressor T lymphocytes, which means that it affected their immune system badly. The whole plant would not have these serious side effects.

In 1999 Guil-Guerrero recommended eating young shepherd's purse leaves in salads since they contain good amounts of sodium, potassium, calcium, magnesium, iron, copper, zinc and manganese, as well as fatty acids, vitamin C, carotenoids and oxalic acid and plenty of fibre.

How to Use

The best way to use the plant is to eat the young leaves as a salad, to benefit from the minerals and vitamins in it. But you can also make a tea from the whole plant (apart from the root) and use it to stop heavy menstrual bleeding and nosebleeds. It is a renowned remedy for flooding during peri-menopause. James Duke recommends taking shepherd's purse tincture after giving birth to help stop bleeding. It contains a protein that acts in the same way as oxytocin, constricting the smooth muscles that support and surround the blood vessels, especially those of the uterus. Other chemicals in the herb may accelerate clotting and still others help the uterus contract, which is why herbalists have recommended using it to help the womb to return to normal size after childbirth. It will also prevent any bacterial infection. Take an infusion of the herb to stop the bleeding of ulcers. It will calm an overactive intestine and help the healing process. *Potter's New Cyclopedia of Botanical Drugs and Preparations* recommends shepherd's purse as a stimulant and diuretic, and to treat chronic diarrhoea. German Commission E recommends shepherd's purse to treat heavy periods and irregular menstrual bleeding, as well as for treating skin injuries.

Dose

Infusion: Steep 30g of shepherd's purse in a pint of boiling water for ten minutes. Drink one cupful of this three times daily.

Liquid extract 1-4 ml (1:1 in 25 % alcohol) three times daily.

Tincture: 1 ml, three times a day.

You can eat the young leaves before it flowers in salads.

Contraindications

Shepherd's purse is not toxic. However, pregnant and lactating women should not take it since it acts like oxytocin and stimulates the uterus to contract.

Chapter 14

Sphagnum moss *Sphagnum spp*

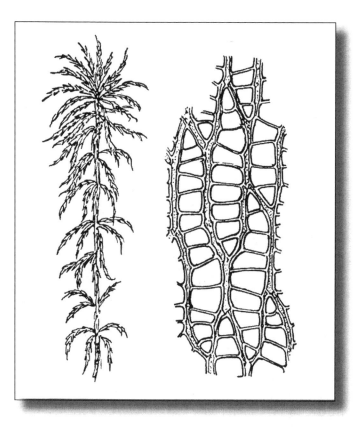

Sphagnum moss covers the moist, rainy hilltops of Wales and Ireland, like a soft, green blanket, sucking up the rain and holding it in its highly absorbent huge hyaline cells. In 1968 Tibbets reported that between one and two per cent of the earth's land surface was covered in peat, built up over thousands of years by layer upon layer of sphagnum, which absorbs enormous amounts of carbon. As the layers of moss die they sink down to form dark layers of peat and new, green layers form on top. It's a slow process, one centimetre taking three hundred years when there is plenty of rain, much longer during dry periods. Sphagnum draws up the water table during high rainfall periods. There are at least three hundred different species of sphagnum moss worldwide, but by far the greatest amount of moss is found in the northern part of the Northern Hemisphere. There are eleven well defined groups of species, of which six grow in Britain. Unfortunately peat bogs are under threat from climate change, acid rain, which has destroyed large areas in the southern Pennines, peat fired power stations in Ireland and garden centres, which sell peat as compost.

Mrs Grieve has a lot to say about sphagnum moss:

A Gaelic Chronicle of 1014 relates that the wounded in the battle of Clontarf 'stuffed their wounds with moss,' and the Highlanders after Flodden stanched their bleeding wounds by filling them with bog moss and soft grass. She says that stricken deer drag their wounded limbs to beds of sphagnum moss; that the Kashmiri have used it from time immemorial. An old writer says: 'The Lapland matrons are well acquainted with this moss. They dry it and lay it in their children's cradles to supply the place of mattress, bolster and every covering, and being changed night and morning, it keeps the infant remarkable clean, dry and warm.' The Lapps also use the moss for surgical purposes, and the Newfoundlanders have been dressing their wounds and sores with it for many centuries. In the nineteenth century, people used sphagnum moss, together with peat fibre, as a rooting medium for orchids, because it retains moisture like a sponge. During the two world wars people collected sphagnum moss in Scotland, Ireland, Wales, Devon, the Yorkshire moors, the Lake District and the Wye Valley so that doctors could dress the wounds of the soldiers. Sometimes the doctors at the front soaked the sphagnum moss in raw garlic juice diluted with water. The Government, recognising the antibiotic qualities of garlic, bought up tons of garlic bulbs and sent them to the doctors treating the wounded.

The Physicians of Myddvai make frequent mention of moss in their recipes, which suggests that the ancient Celts would have used it; and although the Physicians of Myddvai seldom specify which species of moss they used it is likely they would have used sphagnum moss, since there is such an abundant supply of it in Wales.

Botanical Description

Soft, porous, star-like florets grow on the top of the sphagnum stem, which then develops branches that continue to grow, while the main stem of the moss stops growing longer. This results in the branches forming a compact dome-like head. Later the whole plant elongates. Between thirty and one hundred and fifty leaves grow out of each branch in a spiral. The pale-green species is the most common, but there are several others, large and small, varying in colour from very light green to yellow, all shades of pink to deep red and brown. The leaves contain hyaline cells, which are one-cell thick and are unusually large and porous. They live for a year or two, while more branches grow above them, eventually killing them with shade. Layers of dead sphagnum accumulate under living sphagnum as peat. It needs wet, acidic conditions to grow and contains only one per cent nitrogen and very little oxygen or calcium. So it decays very slowly, as does anything thrown into it, which explains why entire bodies of men, such as Lindow Man, found in Cheshire, have been found in peat bogs, preserved intact for thousands of years. Given the right conditions the peat can reach a depth of fifteen metres, but it is usually only one to five metres deep. Relatively high rainfall throughout the year, such as in Ireland and Wales, is ideal for sphagnum, which may blanket the whole countryside. In regions where there is a summer drought it is sometimes localised in basins. Some of the more acid forming species of sphagnum form hummocks, raised above the green carpet of the bog.

Habitat
The highlands of the northern hemisphere where it rains a lot.

Season
Sphagnum moss grows all year round.

Parts Used
The upper layers of the moss.

Preservation
During the two world wars people living near peat bogs, who were too old or too young to fight in the war, trudged out to the bogs to collect the growing plant, with its underlying layers of withered stems and leaves. They squeezed the water out carefully, carried it home in sacks, picked out all the other plants, pine needles, dead insects etc., and separated the strands before spreading it out to dry. They packed the dried moss in muslin bags, two ounces of the moss to each 10 by14 inch bag and sent them to the depots, where they were sterilised.

Although I feel sure that the ancient Celts used sphagnum moss, we are less likely to need to use it today, since we do not have pitched battles with swords and arrows. Our soldiers are treated in well-equipped hospitals.

Properties
Sphagnum moss is, above all, extremely absorbent.

Chemical Constituents
Sphagnum moss contains several different types of sugars: glucose, galactose, arabinose, xylose mannose and ribose, as well as polysaccharides, according to Black in 1955. It also contains amino-acids and 'β'-sitosterol, crude fats, nitrogen and cellulose.

Research

Ancient herbals frequently referred to the use of moss and specifically to sphagnum moss. Tess Darwin said in 1996, 'Sphagnum is the only kind of moss which seems to have been separately distinguished in folk medicine. The abundant remains of *Sphagnum palustre* accompanying a skeleton in a Bronze Age grave in Fife have been interpreted as packing for a wound.' In 1995 Mary Beith said, 'Absorbency of bog moss has been widely valued in Highlands for such purposes as menstrual bleeding and as forerunner of the disposable nappy.' In Ireland people used sphagnum to treat wounds and burns. In Devon people covered the moss with clay.

Chapter 15

Tormentil *Potentilla erecta*

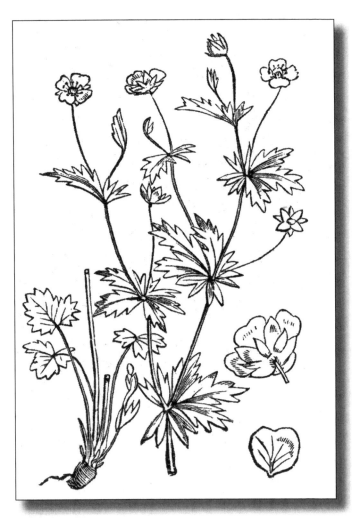

Tormentil (also known as *Potentilla tormentilla*) has been growing in Britain since the last Ice Age and was much used by the
Physicians of Myddvai. In Irish, tormentil is known as Nealfart-
ach: Neal meaning gloom and fartach meaning injury or hurt.

In County Cork the plant is known as Lus an Chodlata: herb for sleep and Neal Codladh: snooze; so it would appear that the ancient Celts used it to make a sleeping draft.

Botanical Description

Tormentil is a low growing, small, perennial plant with a hard root. Its stems are ten to twenty-five centimetres long, some sticking up, some lying flat along the ground. Its stalkless leaves are digitately divided into four or five leaflets with toothed margins and grow up the stem on alternate sides. The leaves are hairy underneath and occur in groups of three with two stipules which look like small leaflets, so there appear to be five leaflets in each group. In summer yellow flowers with four indented petals and many yellow stamens appear in cymes. All other *Potentilla* species have five petals.

Habitat

It grows on acid soils, such as the mountainous bog and moorland and upland meadows of Wales and in dry sandy pinewoods and heathland.

Season

Tormentil flowers from June to September.

How to Grow

Tormentil grows best in full sun, on soils that are fertile and acidic but you can grow it in a dry sandy flower border or rockery where it will attract bees and butterflies. Sow the seeds in spring in sand or compost. Cover lightly and plant out later in the year.

Parts Used

The rhizomes.

Preservation

Dig up the rhizomes in summer or early autumn, remove the roots, scrub them clean, slice them up and dry them in a warm, airy place.

Properties

Aqueous extracts of the fresh tormentil roots are a rich, deep red-brown, indicating that they contain a lot of tannin, or polyhenols, which are astringent and powerfully antioxidant. The British Herbal Pharmacopoeia recommends tormentil for ulcerative colitis and diarrhoea, due to its astringent and anti-haemorrhagic effect. Herbalists today use tormentil for irritable bowel syndrome, colitis, ulcerative colitis, diarrhoea and rectal bleeding.

Chemical Constituents

Tormentil root contains up to twenty per cent tannin: both condensed (procyanidins) and hydrolysable (ellagitannins,) according to Fechka in 2015. The hydrolysable tannins include agrimoniin, pedunculagin and laevigatins, according to Geiger in 1994. It contains, galloylquinic acid and catechin and 1.7% triterpenoid saponins according to Stachurski in 1995, including tormentoside, euscaphic acid, pomolic acid, ursolic acid and rosamultin, according to Kite in 2007 and Bilia in 1992.

Research

In 1994 Vennat investigated the antioxidant effect of procyanidin compounds (condensed tannins) from tormentil and found that the larger compounds were the most effective. In 1996 Bos found that different procyanidins from Tormentil had different antioxidant properties. In 2002 Langmead found that the tormentil extract had an antioxidant effect on inflamed tissue from the human colon. This suggested that it would help allay the symptoms of inflammatory bowel disease.

In 2007 Moss and Chefetz carried out a small study on 16 patients who all suffered from active ulcerative colitis. The patients all continued with their normal medication alongside three doses of tormentil extract each for three weeks with washout periods of four weeks. They found that a dose of 2400 mg was the most effective. Stool frequency and blood in the stool decreased. In 2003 Subbotina carried out a clinical trial in Russia on forty children who were in hospital with diarrhoea caused by rotavirus. He gave the children three drops of tincture per year of age three times a day of either tormentil or a placebo. He made the 1:10 tincture from dried root using 40% ethanol, 60% water. The treatment group was between 4-79 months old and the control group was between 3-60 months old. He gave both groups oral rehydration. The treatment group made a significantly faster recovery. They needed less rehydration, their stool consistency improved faster and they left hospital sooner. For example after forty-eight hours diarrhoea had stopped in 8 out of 20 in the treatment group but in only 1 out of 20 in the control group. The placebo was a tincture of Indian tea. Interestingly in 2006 Palombo investigated traditional medicinal plants used to treat diarrhoea and he found that Indian black tea, which is also used to treat diarrhoea, inhibits the rotavirus that affects cows *in vitro*.

How to Use

Since tormentil root contains such a lot of tannin it is ideal for treating all types of diarrhoea caused by inflammations or infections, such as ulcerative colitis and irritable bowel syndrome, as well as providing relief from enteritis, gastritis and rectal bleeding. Use it to treat excessive menstrual bleeding, rheumatism and gout. It is a valuable remedy for severe burns since it will form an antiseptic shield to protect the burn while it heals.

Make a decoction by boiling the root to use as a gargle and to cure pharyngitis and laryngitis, sore gums and mouth ulcers. Add tormentil decoction to St John's wort, Valerian and hops to induce sleep. You might need to add honey to this in order to be able to drink it! Take a tormentil decoction for heavy periods, especially during peri-menopause. Make a weak decoction to cure conjunctivitis.

Make an ointment by grinding up the dried rhizome and mixing it with a solid fat or oil and beeswax melted together. Use this to treat haemorrhoids, sores and wounds.

Make a tincture by grinding up the dried rhizome or chopping up the fresh rhizome and covering it with a mixture of forty per cent alcohol and sixty per cent water. Some strong vodkas are forty per cent alcohol. Leave to steep for twenty-four hours if you have ground it up, two weeks if it's chopped. Strain through fine muslin or a fine coffee filter and store in glass bottles, away from sunlight. Make a liquid extract by adding ground dried rhizome to a mixture of twenty-five percent alcohol and seventy-five per cent water. Some strong wines, such as port are twenty-five per cent alcohol.

Dose

Make an infusion with 12-18 g dried root (rhizome) in one litre of water, divide this into three portions to drink a portion three times a day between meals.

Make a decoction by boiling 2-3 spoons (8-12g) of dried rhizome in a litre of water.

Mix 4-6 g of dried, powdered root directly with fruit juice or lemon, honey and hot water and drink between meals.

Tincture 2-4 ml 3 times a day between meals.

Liquid extract 2-4 ml 3 times a day between meals.

Capsules of dry extract, 2 capsules 3 times a day, each capsule containing 200mg of dry extract, between meals.

Contraindications

It is not a good idea to use tormentil long term, since the large amounts of tannin in it may inhibit the uptake of protein and iron. In 1996 Haslam showed that tannins combine with proteins and minerals and in 2008 Thankachan demonstrated that people who drank tea with their food did not absorb as much non-haem iron as people who did not drink tea with their food. Never take tormentil together with food, but always between meals. Other herbs such as agrimony and raspberry leaf are more suitable for long-term use because they are less astringent, but they too should be taken between meals.

Chapter 16

Violet *Viola odorata*

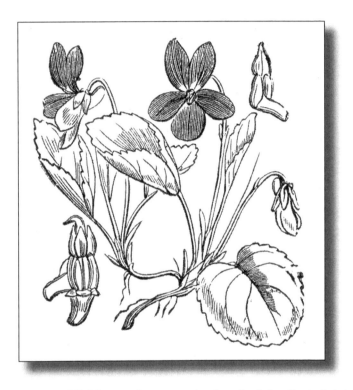

When I was a child I was always excited to find the first violet of spring, after the long, cold winter. I would find it, half hidden, in amongst the muddled vegetation growing on the steep bank of the lane, between the leaves of the not yet flowering plants of primrose, dog's mercury, celandine, grasses, ivy and the gnarled roots of the hedgerows above.

Many years later I stared through the plate glass windows of a bar in Florence at piles of candied violets and rose petals, too expensive to buy. Someone had painstakingly captured the essence of these flowers and embalmed them in sugar. The ancient Salernitan herbal has a recipe for violet sugar, which will keep for three years: one pound of flowers to three to four pounds of sugar, chop the flowers, mix with the sugar in a glass container, place in the sun for three days, stirring every day.

Violet has been growing in Britain since before the last Ice Age and was used by the Physicians of Myddvai, so we can definitely call it a Celtic herb. The early settlers took violet seeds with them to North America, where they spread and made their home.

The ancient Greeks, who considered that violets were a symbol of fertility and love, made them into love potions. People have been presenting bouquets of violets to the beloved throughout the ages. Gerard tells the tale of the 'young demosell, Io, that sweete girle, whom Jupiter courted' then 'he had got her with child'. After she had given birth he turned her into a 'trim heiffer,' according to Dodoens, to protect her from the jealous eyes of Hera. He made violets grow as fragrant food for her. (Small consolation after being raped and turned into a cow!) Since love is associated with the heart and the spurned lover is 'broken hearted', the ancient Greeks gave violet infusions as a tonic for the heart.

Juliette De Bairacli Levy wrote in 1973 that violet flowers and leaves have been used for relaxing and calming deranged nerves. *Viola odorata* is used in the Lebanon as a remedy for influenza, coughing and as a diuretic, expectorant and sedative.

Botanical Description

It is a small, perennial plant with a stout rootstock, found in hedgerows, rough land and margins of woodlands. The leaves grow on stalks in a rosette from the root and are heart shaped and hairy with an oval stipule. The flowers are dark purple or white, have five petals and hang down from a curved stalk. The lowest petal has a prominent nectar-filled spur and the five sepals have basal appendages. It sends out long, creeping stolons, from which fresh plants grow. It has a beautiful, delicate scent.

Habitat

In Britain violet is a hedgerow plant, growing on banks and grass verges of country lanes.

Season

Violets flower in the early spring.

How to Grow

Violets will grow just about anywhere, as long as they do not have to compete with too many other plants. The seeds need to be chilled before they will germinate. This is usually not a problem in Britain, if you sow the seeds in the autumn, since the winter frosts will do the trick. Once the violet plants become established they will spread and take over an area where nothing else is growing. I find them growing in the gravel round my summerhouse! They need water, so the gentle rains of spring in Britain create ideal conditions for them to flourish.

Part Used

Flowers, roots and leaves.

Preservation

Dig up the roots in autumn and dry them. Harvest the flowers and leaves in early spring, dry them in a warm, airy place away from the sun and store in glass jars in a dark place. Make a violet oil by infusing violet flowers in almond oil for two weeks in the sun, straining through muslin and storing in glass containers in a dark place.

Properties

Violet flowers, leaves and roots store a cornucopia of valuable compounds with all sorts of healing properties: The mucilage in violet is soothing and anti-inflammatory, the saponins in the roots are expectorant, the salicylic acid eases pain and brings down a fever and the whole plant is antibacterial. The quercetin and scopoletin in the plant are anti-asthmatic. The rutin in the flowers helps maintain and strengthen the walls of the capillaries, so can help treat varicose veins. *Viola odorata* is diaphoretic, diuretic, laxative, emollient, antipyretic, sedative, antibacterial, antioxidant, protects the liver and lowers cholesterol.

Chemical Constituents

Violet contains flavonoids, including quercetin (in the plant) and generous amounts of rutin (in the flowers). In 1991 Lamaison found 18% mucilage in the flowers in France, then in 2005 Drozdova and Bubenchikov found mucilage in the leaves: mainly galactose, glucose and galacturonic acid. The wild flowers may have 0.003% volatile oil, which has at least 63 different components, including eugenol, linalool, benzyl alcohol, α-canidol, globulol and viridiflorol, zingiberene, according to Bradley and trans-alpha-ionone gives the characteristic fragrance according to Werkhoff in 1991. Violets contain acids, including salicylic, ferulic, sinapic (in the plant) and malic (in the flowers.) They contain alkaloids, including scopoletin (in the plant), odoratine (in the roots) and violin (in the flowers). The roots contain saponins. Violets contain alcohols, including eugenol, and sterols, including beta sitosterol, and vitamins, including vitamins A and C. The root contains about 30 cyclotides, including violacin A, according to Ireland in 2006; these are strange looking compounds with a circular head-to-tail backbone.

Research

There has been a great deal of interest in the medicinal properties of *Viola odorata* but most of the research has been carried out in the laboratory, often in Iran, where violet is used traditionally as a herbal medicine. Several scientists, including Arora in 2007, have demonstrated that all parts of *V odorata* are very effective at killing bacteria. In 2012 Siddiqi and his team demonstrated that extract of violet leaves lowered blood pressure, slowed down the heart rate and reduced cholesterol and triglycerides (bad fats) in the blood of rats who had been fed a high fat diet. In 2010 Ebrahimzadeh and his team found that *V odorata* flowers were antioxidant and scavenged free radicals. In 2009 Kumar and his team showed that violet extracts were diuretic and laxative. In 2013 Monadi and his team demonstrated that violet leaf extract was sedative in rats. In 2013 Elhassaneen and his team found that violet flower powder protected the liver and kidneys. In 2009 Vishala and team demonstrated the laxative effects of *Viola odorata* leaves and flowers. In 1985 Khattak and team showed that violet extracts would bring down a fever in rabbits. In 2006 Amer demonstrated that violet essential oil would repel mosquitoes. In 2003 Koochek demonstrated that *Viola odorata* extract is anti-inflammatory in rats.

Scientists were very excited to discover cyclotides in violet flowers and roots. These compounds are peptides which do not break down when they are heated. Nor do enzymes break them down. Violets create these strange compounds to protect themselves from insects, but they also stimulate the uterus, are anti-HIV, antibacterial, toxic to cells and to haem: the red compound in our red blood cells. In 2010 Gerlach and his team found that a cyclotide from *Viola odorata* had anti-tumour effects on breast cancer cells *in vitro*. They showed that the cyclotide disrupted the membrane of the tumour cell. Interestingly it did not have the same effect on other types of cancer, only on the breast cancer cells. But violets contain at least thirty different cyclotides which could have different anti-cancer effects.

In 2002 Lindholm and team suggested that cyclotides might be used as leads to anti-tumour agents but this is yet another example of the pharmaceutical industry isolating a compound from a plant in the hope that they can make small changes to its structure, patent it and sell it as an expensive drug. Isolated cyclotides are too toxic to use, but within the plant, together with a multitude of other compounds which buffer them, they act as valuable medicine. Herbalists have been using *Viola odorata* for some time to treat cancers, since they have observed that it is sometimes effective, when used in combination with an array of other herbs.

In Iran there have been some clinical trials with violet, including one to demonstrate that violet oil would cure insomnia. Almost a third of the populations in industrialised countries suffer from some kind of sleep disturbance at some point in their lives. Doctors usually prescribe benzodiazepines but the side effects include amnesia, sedation, slowness, sleepiness, fatigue, headache, irritability and dizziness. Violet oil, on the other hand, is a known medication for treating insomnia in Iranian traditional medicine. It is hypnotic and sedative, without the harmful side effects of benzodiazepines. Plants containing antioxidant and polyphenolic compounds protect the nerves and violet contains plenty of these compounds. It contains the hypnotic linalol; and some flavonoids, sterols, alkanes and terpenoids which also have a hypnotic effect. The rutin in violet has a sedative effect while the melatonin in violet is hypnotic and helps to rebalance circadian rhythms. So in 2014 Feyzabady and his team in Iran decided to test violet oil on insomniac patients. They made the violet oil by mixing violet flowers with sweet almonds in 1:2 proportions, then pressing the resultant mixture to extract an almond violet oil, which they stored in dark glass containers. Each millilitre of the oil contained 924 mg of violet oil. They gave the violet oil to 50 chronic insomniacs and told them to put two drops of the oil into their nostrils each night at bedtime for a month. At the end of this period most of the patients said that their sleep had improved. There were a few transient side effects.

In 2015 Qasemzadeh and his team in Iran gave violet syrup or placebo, along with common standard treatments, to 182 children aged 2-12 years, who had a cough and intermittent asthma.

The cough improved in the children who took the violet syrup.

How to Use

Make a calming tea with violet leaves, vervain and elderflower for a calm, restful sleep. Add violet root and plant to your cough mixtures. Take the root decoction to treat bronchitis, rheumatism and arthritis. You can also soak a small towel in the decoction and wrap it around the painful joint or even pour the decoction into your bath. Or make an ointment by heating the leaves in a hard fat or an oil and beeswax mixture. Make an infusion of the flowers, mix with lemon juice and honey and drink three cups a day to treat colds, coughs and influenza. Take an infusion of the flowers to calm your nerves and to reduce the swollen mucous membranes of the bronchi during an asthmatic attack.

Make a tea from the dried flowers to treat gastritis, stomach and duodenal ulcers. The mucilage will have a soothing effect. The anti-inflammatory and analgesic properties will relieve the pain and reduce the inflammation. Take an infusion of the flowers to help get rid of bacteria in the urinary tract, sooth and cool the urethra and cure cystitis. But if the condition persists you must see a doctor. Rub the oil onto your legs to treat varicose veins. Add fresh violets to salads: half a cupful per person is perfectly safe.

Dose

1-2 g of dried flower powder twice a day.

2-4g dried herb three times a day.

Infusion: one tablespoon of dried flowers and/or leaves to a pint of water.

Decoction of root: three tablespoons of chopped, dried violet roots in one litre of water, boiled for twenty minutes. Take 4 tablespoons per day.

Tea from the flowers and leaves, either fresh or dried: one teaspoon of dried herbs to a cup of boiling water or one tablespoon to a pint. Cover and leave to stand for ten minutes, strain and drink three cupfuls a day.

Contraindications

Violets are quite safe but you should be careful not to overdose on the tincture or decoction. Do not take violet during pregnancy or lactation. Only give very small doses to children.

Chapter 17

Watercress *Nasturtium officinale*

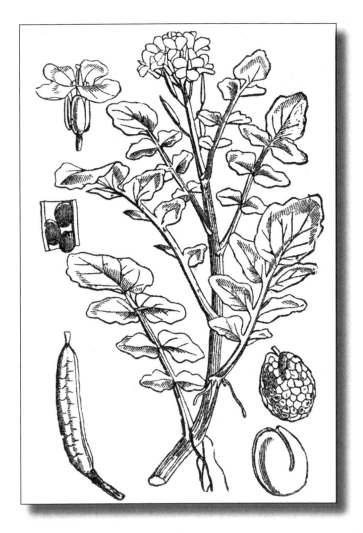

When I was a child we found watercress growing around a spring in the Banky Meadow, its smooth, glossy green leaves inviting us to pick it. But we had been told never to eat it because tiny snails could live hidden amongst its leaves and these snails were the host of the liver fluke, a parasite that infected sheep. This parasite, we were told, could also infect us, burrowing into our livers and making us ill. So we looked longingly at the lovely green leaves and left it where it was.

Hippocrates, the father of western medicine, built his first hospital in Kos, Greece, near a river where he could grow watercress to help treat his patients. He called it the 'cure of cures'. Native to Britain, it is a member of the Cruciferae family and grows happily in the shallow streams and cool pools of Wales, where the ancient Celts would have picked it. Farmers now cultivate it in Britain as well as in North America.

Botanical Description
It has smooth, shiny heart-shaped leaves growing on floating or crawling stems, six leaves opposite each other and one at the end on each stem. Clusters of tiny flowers, four to six millimetres in diameter with four white or pink-white petals, grow at the ends of the stems. Bees love them for they are a rich source of pollen. The trailing stems produce new roots at the leaf nodes and so watercress tends to spread, forming brilliant green mats, where it finds clean, slow flowing, cool water.

Habitat
Shallow streams from chalky hillsides.

Season
Spring, summer and autumn.

How to Grow
Ideally, if you want to grow watercress, you will need a slow flowing stream, preferably coming from chalky or limestone soils; and the stream should not come from fields where livestock live. It is very sensitive to pollution but when it has a pure water source it will grow fast. It prefers to grow in about five

centimetres deep water with an optimum pH of 7.2. But it is possible to grow the plants in wet soil in a shaded position if you protect the plants in winter, but you might end up with very hot flavoured watercress.

Parts Used
The leaves.

Preservation
It is better to eat watercress raw.

Properties
People in Iran have been using watercress as a folk remedy for high blood pressure, hyperglycaemia (high blood sugar levels) and renal colic (kidney pain) for centuries. Herbalists in Britain use watercress as a diuretic, expectorant, digestive and to treat eczema, colds, coughs, renal colic, liver diseases and to improve blood circulation. Recently scientists have discovered anticancer, antiviral, antioxidant, anti-inflammatory and liver protective properties.

Chemical Constituents
Watercress is a rich source of Vitamins C, A, and B complex (thiamine, riboflavin, niacin, pantothenic acid, pyridoxine, biotin and folic acid).

Watercress contains significant amounts of minerals, such as calcium, copper, phosphorous, iron, magnesium, manganese, potassium, sodium, iodine and zinc, according to Bremness in 1994.

Glucosinolates, e.g. gluconasturtin appear to be the main active constituents, and most likely the chemicals responsible for the plant's effectiveness at reducing inflammation and mucous in the nose, throat and bronchi, according to Hecht in 1995. It contains Isothiocyanates, including 2-Phenethyl isothiocyanate, which can reduce carcinogen activation. Carcinogens are substances that can cause cancer, if they are activated. But no one has carried out clinical trials to demonstrate that watercress prevents cancer. It contains amino acids such as beta carotene and phenolic compounds, which are powerfully antioxidant.

Research

Scientists all over the world have carried out a great deal of research into the chemistry of watercress. There have also been plenty of experiments in the laboratory, both on extracts of the whole plant and on compounds isolated from it. For example in 2002 Fekadu Kassie and his team in Austria found that watercress juice protected the DNA in cells from damage. Watercress contains large amounts of gluconasturtin, which breaks down to phenethyl isothiocyanate, which the scientists concluded was responsible for the protective effect. The cells in our bodies are constantly bombarded by toxins and low levels of radioactivity, which can damage their DNA, leading to ill health, including cancer. This research does not prove that eating watercress protects us from cancer but there is a good chance that it might, given that it contains DNA protecting compounds.

In 2004 Peter Rose and his team in the University of Singapore isolated isothiocyanates from watercress. They found that isothiocyanates stopped macrophages (a type of white blood cell) from producing too much nitric oxide and prostaglandins. Excess nitric acid and prostaglandins can cause chronic inflammation so they suggested that isothiocyanates could reduce inflammation. In 2013 Sadeghi and his team in Iran found that watercress extracts significantly reduced the inflammation of rats' paws and mice's ears.

Mousa-Al-Reza Hadjzadeh and his team found that diabetic rats had higher levels of cholesterol and glucose in their blood than rats that were not diabetic. However, after drinking watercress extract for four weeks the diabetic rats' glucose and cholesterol levels went down significantly. This does not prove that watercress will lower cholesterol and glucose in diabetic humans, but there is a chance that it might. In Turkey Tevfik-Zen found that watercress extracts had strong anti-oxidant activity and reduced free radicals. Free radicals damage the cells in our bodies which can cause many diseases, including cancer, atherosclerosis and cellular degeneration related to ageing. Phenolic compounds from plants, such as polyphenols, flavonoids and terpenes protect living cells from free radicals. Watercress is full of phenolic compounds.

In 2013 Freitas and team in Portugal found that combinations of watercress extracts and antibiotic were more powerful against *E coli* bacteria than the antibiotic alone.

Unfortunately there have been few clinical trials with watercress. However, in 2006 Goos and his team in Germany carried out a trial on 858 children, between 4 and 18 years with acute sinusitis, bronchitis or urinary tract infection. They either gave them a herbal preparation of watercress and horseradish or an antibiotic. The patients recorded in a diary when they took the medication and whether they suffered any side effects. The doctors in charge of the patients found that the herbal preparation was just as effective as the antibiotics and the children suffered from fewer side effects. Since the watercress was mixed with horseradish this does not prove that watercress on its own could cure sinusitis, bronchitis or urinary tract infection. Given that watercress contains so many active compounds, more clinical trials are needed.

In 2002 Thomson and Shaw compared the incidence of colorectal cancer in Maori and non Maori people in New Zealand. They were surprised to find that although the Maoris ate more red meat and saturated fat and drank more alcohol than the non-Maoris, almost half as many of them suffered from colorectal cancer. They discovered that the Maoris ate sow thistle (*Sonchus sp*) and watercress (*Nasturtium officinale*) as a regular part of their diet, which could have been responsible for the cancer protective effect, since the non-Maoris did not eat these plants.

The German Commission E approved watercress for catarrh of the respiratory tract. In Germany it is also used to treat urinary tract infections in children, according to Schilcher in 1997.

How to Use
Seek out organic watercress and eat it whenever you can, raw in salads or in sandwiches to protect yourself from diseases such as rheumatism caused by inflammation, to prevent colds, coughs and flu and to help prevent cancer.

Dose
20-30g of fresh herb per day or,
4-6g dried herb per day or,
60-150 ml freshly pressed juice per day.

Contraindications
A few people are allergic to watercress and may suffer dermatitis if they touch the leaves. People suffering from gastric and intestinal ulcers or inflammatory kidney disease should not eat watercress. It's not recommended during pregnancy.

Part III: A Few Poisonous Plants Used by the Celts

The Physicians of Myddvai used many different poisonous plants, such as hemlock (*Conium maculatum*), hellebore (*Heleborus niger*), rue (*Ruta graveolens*), greater celandine (*Chelidonium majus*), elder leaves (*Sambucus niger*), tansy (*Tanacetum vulgare*), broom (*Cytisus scoparius*), ground elder (*Aegopodium podagraria*), water hemlock (*Cicuta douglasil*), dropwort (*Oenanthe spp*), ivy (*Hedera spp*), yew (*Taxus baccata*), bitter night shade (*Solanum dulcamara*), nightshade (*Atropa belladona*) and mandrake (*Mandragora officinarum*). They used some of these plants as emetics, some of them as emmenagogues (or abortifacients), sometimes they made ointments or plasters from them; they even made anaesthetic potions. This suggests that the ancient Celts also used some of these poisonous plants, internally and externally. I have no doubt that they knew how to use poisonous plants to kill, as well as to heal. I have chosen to focus on just three poisonous plants used by the ancient Celts.

Chapter 1

Foxglove *Digitalis purpurea*

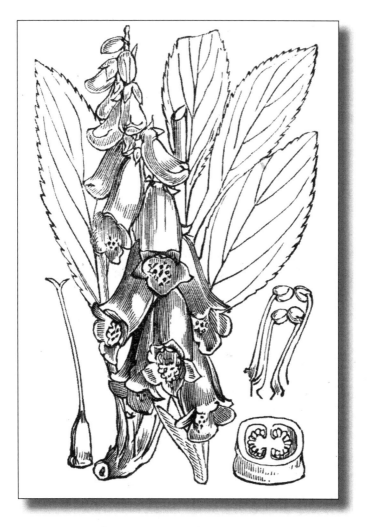

Foxglove was the glove of the good folk or fairies, whose favourite haunts were in the deep hollows and woody dells, where the foxglove delights to grow. Folksglove is one of its oldest names, and is mentioned in a list of plants in the time of Edward III.

There is a northern legend that bad fairies gave these blossoms to the fox so that he could put them on his toes to soften his tread when he prowled among the roosts. The spots on the foxglove and the cowslip, like those on butterfly wings and on the tails of peacocks and pheasants, were the marks where the elves had put their fingers, and one legend says that the marks on the foxglove were a warning sign of the poisonous juices in the plant, which led to the Irish name of Dead Man's Thimbles. People used it as a poison in mediaeval times for 'trial by ordeal'. In Anglo Saxon times Foxes-glees referred to fox music, an ancient musical instrument of bells hanging from an arched support. Leonhard Fuchs (the sixteenth-century herbalist) named the plant *Digitalis* (from *Digitabulum,* a thimble) in 1542 in his *De historia stirpium commentarii.* Fuchs described the plant as a purgative and emetic.

I am including this beautiful but dangerous plant because the Physicians of Myddvai used it in various ways, including internally and because the history of its discovery is so interesting. No one should use foxglove as a medicine today, although it was used medicinally for many years in Britain and various European countries.

Few people knew how to use foxglove as a medicine until Dr Withering discovered it:

> In the year 1775 my opinion was asked concerning a family receipt for the cure of the dropsy. I was told that it had long been kept a secret by an old woman in Shropshire, who had sometimes made cures after the more regular practitioners had failed. I was informed also, that the effects produced were violent vomiting and purging; for the diuretic effects seemed to have been overlooked. This medicine was composed of twenty or more different herbs; but it was not very difficult for one conversant in these subjects, to perceive, that the active herb could be no other than the foxglove.

Dropsy is an accumulation of fluid in the ankles and feet. We now know that it is a symptom of heart failure but in the eighteenth century few people knew this.

The old woman in Shropshire was in fact an illustration by William Meade Prince for an advertising poster for Parke-Davis who marketed Digitalis preparations. So Withering must have got hold of some of this preparation, which he inspected carefully until he identified the active ingredient. Withering was one of those exceptional people who, in addition to being a medical doctor, was also an expert botanist, a chemist and an all round scientist, which explains why he carefully tested the foxglove on turkeys. He went out into the countryside and collected foxglove leaves, stems and roots, and he tested each part of the plant in ever decreasing doses on the unfortunate birds. This was the first instance of toxicology testing. He soon found that the lethal dose was relatively small so he realised that he was dealing with a very powerful plant drug. He decided that in order to measure the correct dose accurately he would have to use only the leaves, collected from second-year plants, just before the first flowers began to appear. He knew that the effect of the leaves might alter at different times of the year and the roots could have a different effect.

After successfully establishing the non lethal dose of dried foxglove leaves for turkeys, Withering went on to treat poor people, free of charge; to all intents and purposes carrying out a large scale clinical trial in a Birmingham hospital. He described the toxic effects of foxglove:

> sickness, vomiting, purging, giddiness, confused vision, objects appearing green and yellow; increased secretion of urine, with frequent motions to part with it; and sometimes inability to retain it; slow pulse, even as slow as 35 in a minute, cold sweats, convulsions, syncope, death.

At first, he, 'thought it necessary to bring on and continue the sickness, in order to ensure the diuretic effects.' As he became more familiar with the drug, however, he modified his practice: 'let it be continued until it either acts on the kidneys, the stomach, the pulse, or the bowels; let it be stopped at the first appearance of any of these effects.' Because of the toxic effects (often delayed) of the leaf decoction, Withering only gave small doses sequentially until either nausea or a diuretic effect was observed and then stopped. Sometimes he added cinnamon or juniper to the composite to hide the disagreeable taste. He was impressed by the diuretic effects of the drug but he also observed that digitalis had: 'a power over the motion of the heart to a degree yet unobserved in any other medicine.' He thought that foxglove might improve 'tumultuous action of the heart' (probably atrial fibrillation) but he did not understand the connection between the heart, dropsy and fluid retention. We now know that digitalin, the active compound in foxglove, inhibits the sodium–potassium pump in cells, so that calcium builds up in the cell. This stimulates the heart muscles to work harder at pumping blood, while slowing down and beating more regularly.

Withering found that the dried powdered leaf was five times as effective as the fresh leaf and was better than a decoction, as boiling seemed to destroy some of the active principle. He then went on to study 163 patients with dropsy, and recorded his results carefully.

One of his reported cases was a Mrs H. of A. The woman, in her forties, exhibited the classic symptoms of severe dropsy. Withering and Darwin found her:

nearly in a state of suffocation, her pulse extremely weak and irregular, her breath very short and laborious, her countenance sunk, her arms of a leaden colour. She could not lie down in bed and had neither strength nor appetite, but was extremely thirsty. Her stomach, legs, and thighs were greatly swollen; her urine very small in quantity, not more than a spoonful at a time, and that very seldom.

Mrs H. was, in fact, so ill that Withering hesitated to prescribe digitalis, fearing that: 'an unfavourable termination would tend to discredit a medicine which promised to be a great benefit to mankind.' But he relented, giving way to 'the desire to save the life of this valuable woman' and prescribed it anyway to marvellous effect. Within a week, every sign of dropsy was gone and Withering reported that she was surviving nine years later, still with occasional bouts of the disease that digitalis fought back every time. Darwin was so impressed that he subsequently wrote perhaps one of the most ponderous and frightfully bad poems ever dedicated to a plant.

In 1785 Dr Withering published his book *Account of the Foxglove*, in which he discussed 158 patients whom he treated with foxglove. Of these, 101 patients with congestive heart failure were cured by the drug, today known as digitalis. He stressed the importance of giving the patient exactly the right dose. But few medical doctors at that time shared his belief in the importance of exact dosage. So after the publication of his book physicians took up the new medicine with enthusiasm, prescribing it for all kinds of conditions where it was ineffective, in too large dosages, with disastrous results. Withering was way ahead of his time and may well have regretted publishing his book when he saw the results. Digitalis fell into disrepute and was not used for many years until histopathology and electrocardiography became established. It was not until 1869 that a French pharmacist, Nativelle, isolated digitalin, the active compound, from foxglove.

Chapter 2

Periwinkle *Vinca minor*

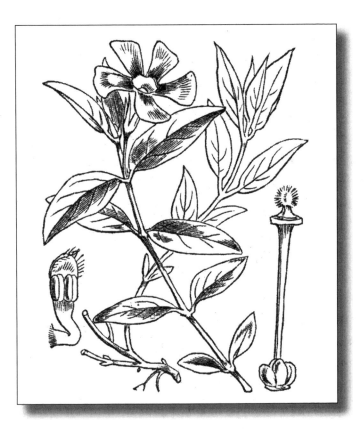

Periwinkle used to grow on the wall that separated our garden from the lane, when I was a child. The lane was lower than the garden, so the wall held up the lawn and the rain seeped into the back of the wall, providing the periwinkle with moisture, so that she could spread her beautiful violet blue flowers out for everyone walking up and down the lane to admire. I think I always knew that this was not a native British plant but it was not until much later that I discovered that the Romans introduced it to Britain. Many centuries later The Physicians of Myddvai used it in their potions. In the eighteenth century, garden centres imported the lesser periwinkle to the United States as an ornamental ground cover. It escaped cultivation and invaded natural areas throughout eastern United States, sometimes forming dense mats on the forest floor, displacing native plant species.

Both the English and botanical names of the Periwinkle are derived from the Latin *vincio* (to bind), since its long, trailing stems spread over and keep down the other plants where it grows. This is described by Wordsworth:

Through primrose tufts in that sweet bower
The fair periwinkle trailed its wreaths.

According to Mrs Grieve the wise folk used Periwinkle to make charms and love-philtres since they believed it had magical properties. It used to be called 'Sorcerer's Violet' ('Violette des sorciers') and was one of the plants people used to exorcize evil spirits. In Macer's Herbal we read of its potency against 'wykked spirytis'. Apuleius, in his Herbarium (printed 1480), said:

This wort is of good advantage for many purposes, that is to say, first against devil sickness and demoniacal possessions and against snakes and wild beasts and against poisons and for various wishes and for envy and for terror and that thou mayst have grace, and if thou hast the wort with thee thou shalt be prosperous and ever acceptable. This wort thou shalt pluck thus, saying, 'I pray thee, vinca pervinca, thee that art to be had for thy many useful qualities, that thou come to me glad blossoming with thy mainfulness, that thou outfit me so that I be shielded and ever prosperous and undamaged by poisons and by water'; when thou shalt pluck this wort, thou shalt be clean of every uncleanness, and thou shalt pick it when the moon is nine nights old and eleven nights and thirteen nights and thirty nights and when it is one night old.

In The Boke of Secretes of Albartus Magnus of the Vertues of

Herbs, Stones and certaine Beastes, we find:

Perwynke when it is beate unto pouder with worms of ye earth wrapped about it and with an herbe called houslyke, it induceth love between man and wyfe if it bee used in their meales ... if the sayde confection be put in the fyre it shall be turned anone unto blue coloure.

Botanical Description

Periwinkle is a trailing, plant, spreading along the ground and sending down roots from its stems to form large colonies and occasionally sending up stems forty centimetres high but never twining or climbing. The leaves are two to four and a half centimetres long, broad, glossy, dark green, leathery, evergreen and grow opposite, each other along the stems. The flowers grow singly in the leaf axils, from early spring to mid-summer, but a few flowers appear in the autumn; they are violet-purple, two to three centimetres in diameter, and the corolla consists of a tubular portion that opens out into a flat disk, composed of five broad irregular petals, twisted when in bud, with unequally curved sides, so that although the whole corolla is symmetrical, when you examine each separate petal you will see that an imaginary line from apex to the centre of the flower would divide it into two very unequal portions.

The mouth of the tube is angular and the tube is closed with hairs, and the curved anthers of the five stamens, are inserted in the tube. The pistil of this flower is a beautiful object, resembling the shaft of a pillar with a double capital. The stigma is on the under surface of the disk, so that the insect's tongue entering the flowers does not cause self-fertilisation.

Habitat

Periwinkle is often found in woods, cemeteries, along roads and other disturbed areas.

Season
Periwinkle flowers in the summer.

How to Grow
Periwinkle will grow in almost any kind of soil: chalk, clay, sand or loam, in full sun or shade, exposed or in a sheltered position. Once it is established it will spread in a dense clump, crowding out every other plant until it meets some obstacle, like a tree or hedge.

Properties
Periwinkle leaves contain high levels of the alkaloid vincamine, which dilates blood vessels and enhances memory. It also has high levels of tannins, so is astringent and bitter.

Chemical Constituents
Scientists have isolated fifty indole alkaloids from the aerial parts and the root of *V. minor,* including vincoside, vincaminorine, vincaminoreine, minovine, minovincine, and vincamine. Vincamine is the dominant alkaloid at 0.057% of the dried plant. It also contains chlorogenic acid.

Research
Vinpocetine is a free radical scavenger that works in a similar way to vitamin E and scientists have carried out numerous studies *in vitro* and *in vivo* on it. Several scientists, including Horvath in 2002 have demonstrated *in vitro* that vinpocetine is antioxidant. Various scientists including Pereira in 2003 and Santos in 2000 have demonstrated *in vitro* and *in vivo* that vinpocetine protects nerve cells from damage caused by lack of oxygen. In 2005 Vas demonstrated that vincamine modulated brain circulation as well as protecting the brain from the harmful effects of lack of oxygen. Vincamine is used to prevent and treat symptoms that result from lack of oxygen to the brain and circulation.

According to Blumenthal there is plenty of clinical evidence that vincamine helps elderly patients with brain disorders, such as memory loss, vertigo, transient lack of oxygen and headache. It increases the flow of blood, oxygen and glucose to the brain which helps it to function better. According to Neuss *Vinca minor* is a natural source for the industrial production of drugs for stimulating blood flow to the brain. In vascular dementia arteries supplying blood to the brain develop atherosclerotic plaques and gradually become blocked. In 1996 Fischhof demonstrated in a double-blind trial that vincamine benefited people with Alzheimer's disease and vascular dementia. One double-blind study found that high amounts of vinpocetine (60 mg per day) had a beneficial effect on hearing loss due to ageing. In 2001 Kolarov assessed the therapeutic effect of vinpocetine on menopausal complaints in three groups of women: a control group of thirty, a second group of thirty-two, with normal amounts of cholesterol in their blood, and a third group of twenty-nine with high levels of cholesterol in their blood, all in early menopause. He found that the menopausal symptoms of the women in groups two and three, who took five milligrams of vinpocetine (Cavinton) three times a day for three months, decreased significantly by the last day of the trial. The women in group three had far less cholesterol in their blood by the end of the trial. In 2000 Truss demonstrated that vinpocetine could be used to treat people suffering from urge incontinence for whom standard medication did not work.

In 1976 Ribari carried out a preliminary study giving ethyl-apovincaminate (a *Vinca* alkaloid) to patients with tinnitus. Tinnitus is caused by lack of blood flow to the inner ear. Ethyl-apovincaminate increases blood flow to the inner ear so he concluded that it might reduce symptoms of tinnitus.

In 2001 Gulyas gave patients who had suffered a stroke a single-dose intravenous infusion of vinpocetine. Then he studied the blood and glucose flow to the brain. He found that more glucose went into the whole brain, as well as to the area affected by the stroke. Numerous studies show that vinpocetine modifies the way the brain uses glucose in acute stroke patients suffering from lack of oxygen to the brain. It also modifies the way the brain uses glucose in chronic stroke patients, particularly in the part of the brain affected by the stroke. In 2005 Szilagy investigated the effect of vinpocetine on forty-three patients with ischemic stroke in a double-blind, randomized, placebo-controlled study. They were suffering from lack of oxygen to the brain. He gave patients either a single dose of twenty mg of intravenous vinpocetine or 500 ml saline as placebo. He found that blood and oxygen to the brain increased in the area affected by the stroke in the patients who received the vinpocetine.

Many scientists have been interested in the anti-cancer potential of *Vinca minor*. In 1988 Proksa demonstrated that vincarubine was cytotoxic to leukaemia cells.

Although scientists have carried out a great deal of research on individual compounds from *Vinca minor*, there has been very little research into the medicinal properties of the whole plant. According to Hoffmann it is a helpful remedy for diarrhoea, bleeding gums and excessive menstrual bleeding and European herbalists have used periwinkle for headaches, vertigo, and poor memory since medieval times.

Use

Herbalists recommend *Vinca minor* for Alzheimer's disease, bleeding gums, bleeding piles, diarrhoea, dizziness, gastric catarrh, headache, heavy menstruation, impaired memory, indigestion and flatulence, loss of hearing, Meniere's disease, nosebleeds, piles and tinnitus. They use it to treat cancer. But you should not use it unless a trained herbalist has given it to you to take. This is why I have not included the dose or the parts used.

Contraindications

Periwinkle should really only be prescribed by a herbalist since it contains toxic vinca alkaloids which can cause nerve, liver and kidney damage if you exceed the prescribed dose and/or if you take the herb over a long period.

Chapter 3

Opium Poppy *Papaver somniferum*

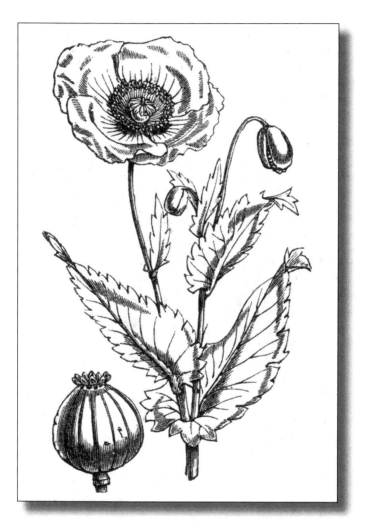

No one knows how long people in the countries where the opium poppy grows have been using it as medicine. 4000 years ago the Sumerians carved images of the poppies and the ancient Minoans knew how to make opium. By the sixteenth century European travellers to the Middle East and India were reporting that people in the Middle East took it as a stimulant, especially when they needed Dutch courage. 'There is no Turk who would not buy opium with his last penny,' the French naturalist Belon noted, 'because they think that they become more daring, and have less fear of the dangers of war.' The Kutch horsemen in Western Gujerat shared their opium with their tired horses, who could then ride further before dropping from exhaustion. In India, John Fryer reported in the 1670s, wrestlers took it to help them to perform feats ordinarily beyond their strength, and warriors, 'to run up on any enterprise with a raging resolution to die or be victorious'. So there is nothing new about athletes taking drugs to improve their performance!

Doctors and healers valued the healing qualities of opium throughout the Mediterranean world for thousands of years. In Lebanon healers used opium to quiet excitable people, to relieve toothache, headache, incurable pain, and for boils, coughs, dysentery and itches and in Algeria people stuffed opium into tooth cavities. When the Roman soldiers at Golgotha took pity on their prisoner on the cross, they added poppy juice to the sour wine they gave him. Jewish authorities say that the plant was well known among the Hebrews more than 2,000 years ago, although the Jerushalmi warns against opium eating, according to Duke. In Arabian countries where doctors practised Unani medicine, they recognised that opium poppy was hypnotic, narcotic, and perhaps harmful to the brain, again according to Duke.

Opium spread northwards from the Mediterranean, transported by traders, to other European countries, including Britain. The ancient Celts who lived along the south coast of Britain before the Romans invaded, imported opium poppy seeds, possibly to use in their cooking. The Physicians of Myddvai used poppies as medicine, so it is likely that the ancient Celts imported opium for its medicinal properties.

The opium poppy, whose Latin botanical name means the

'sleep-bringing poppy', is the king of medicinal plants, containing a veritable cornucopia of active compounds, which can be used by health professionals for a multitude of medical needs. The World Health Organisation lists medicines derived from the opium poppy as essential drugs, because they provide the most effective pain relief.

Botanical Description

The opium poppy is an annual or biennial plant which grows up to one hundred and fifty centimetres. The stem and leaves are sometimes sparsely covered with coarse hairs, sometimes smooth; the stems are slightly branched, with numerous large erect leaves, ovate to oblong, with toothed edges, clasping the stem at the base. The flowers grow on long stalks with nodding buds that expand into magnificent erect flowers with four to eight petals 5-7 cm long, that can be white, purplish, pink, violet, bluish, or red. The fruit is a round or oval, smooth capsule, 4-6 cm long, 3.5-4 cm in diameter, topped with twelve to eighteen radiating stigmatic rays. The seeds are oily, white, dark grey to black, or bluish. The opium poppy flowers and fruits almost throughout the year in tropical areas, elsewhere in spring and summer. All parts of the plant exude white latex when wounded.

The Opium Wars

The opium poppy may have done as much damage to humanity as good, due to its addictive properties, but not until the eighteenth century when, during one of the most infamous periods in British history, the British exported opium to China. At the beginning of the eighteenth century the British East India Company began exporting small amounts of opium from India. Then following the Emperor of China's 1729 edict forbidding the import of opium, the East India Company sold its opium to the owners of merchant ships, who smuggled it into China.

In 1772 Warren Hastings took over the management of the East India Company and increased opium production. By 1830 the East India Company was selling over two million pounds worth of opium to China a year. By March 1839 the Chinese government was so fed up with the opium trade that they confiscated and destroyed more than twenty thousand chests of opium from a warehouse at Canton and blockaded the Pearl River. British warships destroyed the Chinese blockade, took Canton in May 1841, captured Nanjing (Nanking) in August then occupied several Chinese ports and re-opened the opium trade. The British then blocked the entry to the Grand Canal at Zhenjiang, which prevented goods from the southern regions of China from reaching the northern capital. This forced the Chinese to sign the iniquitous Nanking Treaty on the 29th August 1842: the treaty stated that the Chinese had to pay Britain 21,000,000 silver dollars, open several Chinese ports to trade and cede Hong Kong to the British.

In the mid-1850s Chinese officials boarded a British ship in Canton, arrested several Chinese crew members and allegedly lowered the British flag. The British retaliated by bombarding Canton and the Chinese retaliated by burning some British warehouses. The French joined the British, and together they captured Canton in 1857. The same year the British Government took over from the East India Company, Warren Hastings became the first Governor-General of British India and the Opium Act gave the Indian Government a monopoly of the opium trade. In April 1858 the British once again forced the Chinese into negotiations and legalised the importation of opium, then withdrew from Tianjin. When they returned in June 1859 the Chinese shelled them from shore batteries and drove them back with heavy casualties. The Chinese refused to ratify the treaties, so in August 1860 the allies destroyed the Chinese batteries. Then in September they captured Beijing, plundered and burned the emperor's summer palace and forced the Chinese to sign the Beijing Convention, in which they agreed to observe the treaties of Tianjin.

Mass addiction in China reached a level never equaled by any nation before or since. By 1906, twenty-seven per cent of adult Chinese men were addicted. The India-China opium trade ended in 1919 but by then China was producing enough opium to keep the people addicted. In the 1920s, Chiang Kai-shek used the drug cartels to crush Communist labour unions. After Mao Tse-tung's victory in 1949, the Chinese drug cartels fled en masse to Hong Kong and by the 1970s Hong Kong had become a major supplier of heroin to the US market.

Opium consumption in Britain in the nineteenth century

The British Pharmacopoeia Tincture of Opium, or Laudanum, was made with three ounces of opium and equal parts of distilled water and alcohol. In nineteenth-century Britain anyone could buy laudanum cheaply at the chemists and many people did, including the poets Keats, Shelly and Byron. Laudanum was cheaper than beer or wine and even the lowest-paid worker could afford it. Throughout the first half of the nineteenth century, opium addiction increased steadily in England, Europe and the United States and people even gave opium sedatives to children.

In 1874 chemists used acetic anhydride, along with about five other chemicals, to transform morphine into diacetylmorphine (heroin) which is twice as potent as morphine. This became the doctors' drug of choice for severe pain relief. The British Royal College of Anaesthetists adopted the flower and fruit of the opium poppy on their coat of arms in 1992, when they were awarded their Royal Charter.

How to Grow

Opium poppies like a rich, well-manured, deep, warm, moderately moist, medium heavy soil, well cultivated, limed and neutral to slightly alkaline. Grow from seed and thin the plants out so that they stand about 60 cm apart. In Britain we grow opium poppies for their magnificent display, since they hardly produce any opium. They need a hotter climate for that.

Chemical Constituents of Poppy Seeds

Poppy seeds are very nutritious since 100 g contains 533 calories, 18.0 g protein, 44.7 g fat, 23.7 g carbohydrate, 6.3 g fibre, 1,448 mg calcium, 848 mg phosphorous, 9.4 mg iron, 21 mg sodium, 700 mg potassium, 0.95 mg thiamine, 0.17 mg riboflavin, and 0.98 mg niacin. They also contain minute amounts of iodine, manganese, copper, magnesium, sodium, zinc, lecithin, oxalic acid, pentosans, traces of narcotine and an amorphous alkaloid; and the enzymes diastase, emulsin, lipase, and nuclease.

Chemical Constituents of Opium

Opium poppy farmers make cuts on the green seed pods, the latex then oozes from the incisions and they collect it and dry it to produce 'raw opium'. Opium contains about 8-14% morphine, one of the morphinane alkaloids, which include codeine and thebaine. Opium also contains numerous other alkaloids including the pthalide-isoquinoline alkaloids, noscapine and narcotoline and the benzylisoquinoline alkaloids, papaverine and noscapine.

Properties

Opium is analgesic, anodyne, suppresses cough, is anaphrodisiac, astringent, bactericidal, calming, carminative, soothing, emollient, expectorant, stems the flow of blood, lowers blood pressure, is hypnotic, narcotic and sedative. Doctors use its derivatives, morphine, diamorphine and codeine to relieve pain and calm anxiety. It is astringent so sometimes used for diarrhoea. It is expectorant, diaphoretic, sedative and antispasmodic so has been used in cough medicines, though less so these days. Very small doses of opium are stimulant. Opium is not calming and hypnotic for animals but it can be used locally to soothe pain and spasm.

Warning

All opium products, apart from poppy seeds, are restricted to professional doctors, who may only prescribe in cases of severe pain. Opium derivatives are very addictive and should only be used where the pain is short term or the patient is suffering from a terminal disease.

Part IV: The Roman Invasion

Julius Caesar said, 'I knew that in almost all of our campaigns in Gaul our enemies had received reinforcements from Britain.' So, in 55 BCE, he decided to invade Britain and deal with this threat. When the Celtic tribes in Kent saw Caesar's ships approaching, they rushed down to the shore, plunged into the sea and began fighting the Romans before they had time to reach the beach. Caesar said, 'The Romans were faced with serious problems. These dangers frightened our soldiers who were not used to battles of this kind, with the results that they did not show the same speed and enthusiasm as they usually did in battles on dry land.' Later his ships were hit by a sudden storm, which destroyed many of them. He retreated back across the Channel, but not before he had made Commius King of the Atrebates. The Atrebates were a Celtic tribe originally from Gaul, living on the south coast of England in the area around modern-day Chichester in Sussex. A year later Caesar returned and, using Commius as a mediator, managed to establish a base in Britain and deal with the other 'unruly tribes'. He stayed in Britain less than a year, returning to Gaul to quell yet another rebellion.

On the 31st July 2012 Maeve Kennedy reported in the *Guardian* that Michael Fulford and Amanda Clarke, from the Department of Archaeology at Reading University, had discovered an Iron Age town called *Calleva Atrebatum*, while excavating the ancient Roman town of Fishbourne, near modern-day Chichester. *Calleva Atrebatum* means the wooded place of the Atrebates and was Commius the Gaul's base. The town they discovered predated the Roman town by one hundred years. Fulford and Clarke analysed the seeds they found and came to the conclusion that the Atrebates enjoyed a lifestyle similar to that of the Romans, which is hardly surprising since, as already mentioned, they had been trading indirectly with Rome for some time and after Caesar's invasion their links with Rome increased. They ate shellfish, beef, mutton, pork, domesticated birds such as chicken and geese as well as wild fowl, wheat, apples, blackberries, cherries and plums. They used poppy seeds, coriander, dill, fennel, onion, celery and olives, none of which were native to Britain. They imported wine and olive oil in large quantities.

They minted coins with Latin inscriptions, adopted Roman customs, even Roman religious rites. *Caleva Atrebatum* had paved streets, drainage, shops, houses and workshops. A picture was beginning to emerge of Roman influenced Celtic tribes along the southern coast of Britain, before the Romans invaded. It is likely that the Atrebates used and possibly grew medicinal herbs imported from Rome and this may have applied to other Celtic tribes along the southern coast.

In 45 CE, almost one hundred years after Caesar had invaded Britain, Claudius sent his general Vespasian to invade the island. He defeated the Britons near Rochester and marched his forces west, capturing oppida (Celtic hill top settlements) as he went, eventually reaching Exeter. In 54 CE Nero became Emperor and sent his general, Gaius Suetonius Paulinus, to invade Wales, where he encountered fierce resistance. The Celtic tribes in Wales were independent, tough and resistant to tax collectors and fought Suetonius, as he battled his way across from East to West. It took him a long time to reach the North West coast and in 60 CE he finally crossed the sea to the sacred island Mona, or Anglesey, the last stronghold of the Druids. His soldiers attacked the island and massacred the Druids, men, women and children, destroyed the shrine and the sacred groves and threw many of the sacred standing stones into the sea.

This was the point at which everything started to go wrong for the Romans. While Paulinus and his troops were rampaging and massacring Druids in Anglesey, Roman officials the other side of the country in modern-day Essex were behaving badly. The Icenian King, Prasutagus died in 60 CE, leaving a will in which he made Nero and his two daughters co-heirs to his kingdom in modern-day East Anglia. Boudicca, his widow, crowned herself Queen and started to rule. The Romans in charge of the area moved into her kingdom as soon as her husband was buried and divided it up among themselves, then raped her daughters and flogged Boudicca in public. This exemplified the Roman attitude towards women, especially women of conquered tribes. A statue from Aphrodisias in Turkey, which shows Claudius raping a helpless Britannia, demonstrates the Roman attitude towards the lands it conquered and the women in them. Roman women too were subjugated, powerless and kept at home. Celtic women, on the other hand, were fiercely independent, and used to being treated as equals with men.

Miranda Aldhouse-Green describes in her book, *Boudica Britannia*, how a furious Boudicca mounted her chariot with her daughters and drove round the villages and settlements of her kingdom, rallying her troops. We have all seen pictures, if not the actual statue on the Thames embankment in London, of her standing proudly in her chariot with her daughters. Miranda Aldhouse-Green talks of the statues of women with spears, daggers and swords which attest to the fact that Boudicca was a typical Celtic woman warrior. Her people were already angry: angry with the Romans for pushing them off their land and away from their ancestors, angry that the Romans taxed them and imposed their temples and Roman gods and now I imagine that they were angry that their queen had been so publicly humiliated. And so they armed themselves with their long swords, climbed onto their chariots and followed her in a great, shouting, unruly rabble. She led her people out of her kingdom to the Roman city at modern-day Colchester. The downtrodden Celts in this city were furious with the Romans, for taxing them to the bone in order to build a temple to Claudius, so they joined Boudicca's rebellion. Together they sacked, looted and burned the city, smashing the hated temple and destroying the graves of Roman soldiers. Boudicca left the smoking ruins of Colchester and led her ever growing mass of people to London, which they similarly sacked, looted and burned, then on to St Albans which suffered the same fate.

Seutonius Paulinus, hearing of this disaster, marched his troops back from Anglesey, arriving in time to see London burn to the ground. He chose not to intervene but planned the best place to confront Boudicca, who he succeeded in defeating, but not before she had destroyed the three most important Roman cities in Britain. After the battle he sent his troops out to hunt down all the members of the tribes that had surrendered, and murdered great numbers of them. The Roman army burnt the Icenian settlements and the Iceni took centuries to return to their former levels of population. After this Seutonius Paulinus was sent back to Rome and given a desk job to keep him out of harm's way. Then the Romans withdrew from most of Wales, leaving the Celtic tribes there and in Scotland alone. Although the Romans had succeeded in invading Wales, they never conquered the Welsh Celts. Their influence in Wales was transitory and the Celts continued to speak their language and maintain their ancient customs and religion.

By 100 CE things had calmed down in Roman occupied Britain and back on the South Coast, near modern-day Chichester, West Sussex, the Romans built Fishbourne palace right on top of the old Celtic town of *Caleva Atrebatum*. They created a rectangular garden with hedge-lined paths and diverted streams to create ornamental fountains and fill baths. This was alien to the Celts, for whom rivers, lakes and streams were sacred and were to be preserved unchanged. The Romans brought seeds with them from the Mediterranean and planted onions, garlic, chives, lavender, Roman thyme, wormwood, sage, aniseed, fennel, mustard and bay. They stayed in Britain for four hundred years, during which time the local Celts adopted many of the plants that the Romans had introduced to Britain. Several centuries after the Romans had left, the Physicians of Myddvai were still using a number of these Mediterranean plants. I decided to investigate some of these plants in addition to those that were growing in Britain before the arrival of the Romans.

.

Part V: A Few of the Medicinal Plants Introduced by the Romans and Used by the Ancient Celts

Chapter 1

Celery *Apium graveolens*

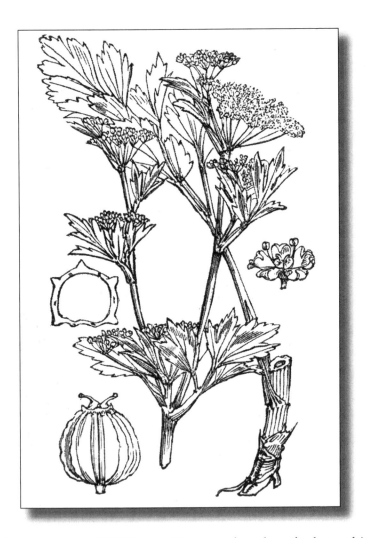

In the summer of 1977 I was sitting on the edge of a long, thin plinth in the consulting room of a herbalist in Wimbledon, surrounded by earnest herbal students and their teacher. I was thirty-two. I told them about the rheumatism that I'd been suffering from for the last four years, ever since I spent the winter in the dampest house imaginable in Chianti Classico. The damp rose up the walls from the river running under the house to meet the wet coming down the walls from the leaking roof above. I developed acute rheumatism in all my major joints, my wrists, elbows, shoulders, hips and worst of all, my knees. The herbal students made up a mixture of herbal tinctures, which included celery seed and dandelion root. I do not remember what the other ingredients were but the celery seed and dandelion root were included specifically to treat the rheumatism. After four months I was cured and I have remained cured ever since.

According to Harry Godwin wild celery is one of a list of species that first appeared in pollen records in the Roman era. The list is a long one and gives us some idea of how many plants may have been introduced by the Romans. Some species were probably survivors from pre-Roman times now finding an opportunity to multiply by forest clearances; others may have been introduced with crops by the Romans. But many plants were deliberately brought to Britain and cultivated. We can find wild celery growing on coastal grassland and the edges of fields.

The ancient Greeks and Romans dedicated celery to Hades/ Pluto, the god of the underworld. They ate it at funeral meals, strewed it on graves and made it into wreaths for the dead. The Greek expression 'deisthai selinon' to need celery, meant that someone had just died. The ancient Greeks and Romans wreathed the victors of their games with celery: a double symbolism of death and victory. Pelikan said, 'Near Selinunt stood the temple of a chthonic underworld god called Apius to whom celery was dedicated.' In ancient Europe people believed that celery would ward off evil spirits. The Physicians of Myddvai used celery as a diuretic, amongst other things, so it is very likely that the ancient Celts began to use it after the Roman invasion.

Botanical Description

The first thing to say about wild celery is that it is a member of the Umbelliferae, a plant family that contains several poisonous species such as hemlock and giant hogweed, so it's not really a good idea to go looking for wild celery, just in case you happen to pick the wrong plant, which would, of course be deadly. It is fine to use the celery that is grown as a vegetable, as long as it is organic.

Wild celery has solid, grooved upright stems and can grow up to one metre tall. It has a shallow tap root system and the stem is branched, succulent and ridged. It has shiny branched leaves each branch of which ends in three pointed leaflets, rather like daggers, two to four and a half cm long. The leaves have short stalks or no stalks and are sheathed by a shiny petiole. In summer they produce small white flowers, in compound umbels, similar to those of cow parsley. Each tiny flower has five petals.

From the 1500s plant breeders selected milder forms of celery to grow as a vegetable in France and Italy, according to Vaughan and Geissler. And according to Sturtevant people were eating it in Britain by the 1700s. Herbalists these days use the common vegetable celery, which is available in shops and supermarkets everywhere.

Habitat

Wild celery is native to Southern Europe and North Africa and grows in marshy areas near or on the coast, including the upper limits of salt marshes and wetlands behind beaches, on coastal grassland and the edges of fields.

Season

In Southern Europe celery is a winter crop but in Britain it is a summer crop.

How to Grow

Celery likes fertile soil, cool temperatures and constant moisture. Soak the seeds overnight before planting them indoors eight to ten weeks before the last frost. Harden off the seedlings before transplanting by reducing water slightly and keeping them outdoors for a couple of hours a day. Work well rotted manure or compost into the ground before transplanting the seedlings ten to twelve inches apart in May. When you dig the plants up be careful to remove every little piece of root since compounds in the root will stop lettuce planted in the same spot from germinating.

Parts Used

Seeds, herb and root.

Preservation

Collect the seeds when they are fully ripe and dry in a warm, airy place away from the sun. Store in an airtight container away from the light.

Properties

The British Herbal Pharmacopoeia, 1983, records that celery seed is anti-rheumatic, sedative and a urinary antiseptic. It's recommended for rheumatism, arthritis, gout and inflammation of the urinary tract. It is potentiated by dandelion root, *Taraxacum officinale*. Celery seed is a mild diuretic and helps to flush away the uric acid crystals that build up around joints or collect in the kidneys to form kidney stones. It also helps to bring down high blood pressure. It is carminative, so eases stomach ache due to flatulence. It is a tonic, good for nervous conditions and helps to promote sleep. It lowers cholesterol, triglycerides and low density lipoproteins (bad fats), so protects the blood vessels from plaque and helps to prevent cardiovascular disease. It is antioxidant and anti-inflammatory and helps to prevent gastric ulcers. It is antifungal.

Chemical Constituents

Celery Seed

Many different scientists including Lin in 2007 Halim in 1990, Kittajima in 2003, have investigated the chemical constituents of celery. Celery seed contains carbohydrates, flavonoids, including the antioxidant apigenin and luteolin; alkaloids, sterols: including deoxy-brassino steroids, which are plant hormones; and glycosides. It has up to 2.45% volatile oil, 60-80% of which is limonene, a compound with many healing properties, including anti-cancer, antioxidant and free radical scavenging; and about 20% is selinene. The volatile oil also contains a large number of other compounds, including caryophyllene, linalool, sedanolide, carvone, and thymol, several of which are antioxidant and anti-inflammatory. It contains tannins, triterpenes, sesquiterpene glucosides; celerioside A-E, isoquercitrin; and phthalides: sedanenolide, sedanolide and sedanonic anhydride, which have many healing properties and mainly account for the characteristic smell of celery. It contains petroselenic, oleic, linoleic, linolenic and palmitic fatty acids. Celery contains furanocoumarins, including bergapten, xanthotodin and isopripinellin.

Celery Herb

Many different scientists including Deng in 2003, Lin in 2007, Kurobayashi in 2006, have identified an array of compounds with healing properties in celery. It contains minerals: magnesium, silica, sodium, potassium, iron, calcium; and vitamins: B6, A and C. It is rich in beta-carotene and folic acid. It contains volatile oil, which is composed of many compounds, including limonene, myrcene, pinene, humulene, ocimene and beta caryophyllene. It contains flavonoids, including luteolin and the anti-inflammatory apigenin; triterpenoids and celerin, bergapten, apiumoside, apiumetin, seddanenolide, cellulose, pectic polysaccharides and sterols. In 2006 Kurobayashi found that the chemical constituents of celery changed when it was cooked.

Celery Root

Celery root contains essential oil: composed of many compounds, including limonene, p-cymene and beta-selinene, which inhibit other plants growing in the same soil and furanocoumarins, which inhibit certain pathogens that infect some vegetables. One furanocoumarin, psoralen, stops lettuce seeds from germinating, according to Bewick in 1994. It contains polyacetylenes which kill cancer cells, according to Zidorn in 2005. It contains carbohydrates, caffeic acid, ferulic acid, coumarin, scopoletin and aescoumelic acid.

Research

As populations in the West are living longer and longer, joint problems have become epidemic. There has been a great deal of research into the anti-inflammatory properties of celery plant and seed. Many scientists, including Lewis in 1985 and Mencherini in 2007, have demonstrated that celery leaf extract is anti-inflammatory. Mencherini isolated apiin, and he found that both apiin and the extract stopped white blood cells from producing nitric acid, which causes inflammation. According to James Duke celery seed contains twenty-five anti-inflammatory compounds, including phthalides and flavonoids.

High levels of uric acid can form crystals in the big toe, instep, ankle, knee, wrist, elbow. This can cause gout, rheumatism and rheumatoid arthritis. Uric acid crystals can also collect in the kidneys to form kidney stones. We all have a certain amount of uric acid in our blood because it is a byproduct of cells breaking down and because food contains elements that form into uric acid. But when we drink too much alcohol or eat too much food containing purines, such as meat, sardines, anchovies, herring, mackerel and scallops our uric acid levels rise if our kidneys can't eliminate it fast enough. Doctors tend to prescribe allopurinol to patients suffering from gout, which stops the production of uric acid but it can upset the stomach, cause skin rash, decrease white blood cells and damage the liver.

Celery seed, on the other hand, does not have these side effects. Several flavonoids from celery seeds reduce uric acid (in mice), according to Shi-Fu in 2007. And it contains 3-n-butylphthalide (3nB), which may inhibit xanthine oxidase, an enzyme involved in the production of uric acid in the liver. There have not been any large scale clinical trials with celery seed to demonstrate that it cures gout or rheumatoid arthritis but many naturopaths and the famous ethnobotanist James Duke all believe that it prevents the buildup of uric acid and cures gout and rheumatism.

Several scientists, including Al-Howiriny in 2010, and Baananou in 2013, have investigated the anti-ulcer properties of celery in rats. Al-Howiriny found that celery herb and seed extracts protected the gut wall from developing ulcers, reduced ulcers that were already there and helped the gut wall to grow new cells to replace those that were damaged by the ulcers. In 1999 Butters registered a patent in the US for the use of celery seed extract to prevent and treat inflammation, pain and gastrointestinal irritation. Again no clinical trials actually prove or disprove that celery prevents and cures ulcers in humans, but the fact that it contains a large number of anti-inflammatory compounds and that it relaxes the walls of the gut suggests that it may well do.

Several scientists, including Baananou have demonstrated that celery extract is anti-bacterial and anti-fungal. In 2002 Friedmen demonstrated that celery seed essential oil kills *Campilobacter jejuni*, a common bacterium found in poultry which can cause reactive arthritis. In 2001 Momin isolated sedanolide and senkyunolide from celery seeds and demonstrated that they killed mosquito larvae, nematodes and funghi, including *Candida*. In 2004 Tuetun found that celery seed extracts repelled mosquitoes from volunteers' skin without irritating it. Active ingredients from celery seed kill nematodes, fungi and insects.

People use celery in Iranian traditional medicine to treat many different conditions, including liver complaints, so in 2007 Taher in Isfahan decided to investigate how the volatile oil extracts of *Apium graveolens* seeds affected liver enzymes in rats. His study showed that D-limonene and myrcene from celery extract stabilise liver cell membranes and thus protect the liver from damage (in rats).

Several different scientists, including Tsi in 2006 and Popovic in the same year, have demonstrated that celery herb extract reduces cholesterol, triglycerides and LDL (bad fats) *in vitro* and *in vivo*. Popovic also demonstrated that celery herb and root extracts scavenge free radicals and inhibit the oxidation of fats. In 2008 Cheng showed that celery seed extract reduces bad fats in the bloodstream and helps to clean up free radicals. This suggests that celery may help prevent fatty plaques from sticking to the walls of the blood vessels, so contributing to the prevention of cardiovascular disease. In 1991 Ko found that apigenin, a major flavonoid from celery plant, relaxes the aorta (the main artery of the body) of a rat. It stopped adrenaline from making the blood vessel contract. If this also applied to humans, celery would help to prevent high blood pressure which contributes to cardiovascular disease.

Male infertility due to low sperm count is a common problem and most of the chemical drugs used to treat it have serious side effects. Celery contains many antioxidant compounds which may protect sperm from damage, and plant hormones which may help to increase male fertility. According to Kerishchi in 2011, celery seed increases testosterone production. Madkur in 2012 demonstrated that celery protects the testes from damage. In 2014 Kooti demonstrated that when he fed celery leaf extract to male rats they produced more sperm. He thought this was partly because celery seed increases testosterone production, which in turn stimulates the testes to produce more sperm. He also thought that the anti-inflammatory flavonoids and phenolic compounds in the celery could have protected the sperm that had already been produced. Celery also contains vitamins E and C, which improve sperm production. There have not been any clinical trials to prove that celery improves male fertility in humans but it is possible that it might.

Several scientists have applied for patents for celery extracts to treat a number of different conditions including: prevention of hair loss during the menopause (Blaszkowski 2008) and prevention of bone loss during menopause (Van Helvoort 2002). Celery contains phytoestrogens which may help to alleviate the symptoms of menopause, but again there have been no clinical trials to prove or disprove this.

Doctors prescribe sodium valporate to treat epilepsy and other diseases. Unfortunately it has severe toxic effects on the testes. So in 2014 Kooti demonstrated in the laboratory that pre-treatment with celery seed extract reduces most of the side effects of sodium valporate.

Properties

Celery stalks and seed are powerfully anti-inflammatory. Celery stops the immune system from producing inflammatory nitric acid, reduces uric acid crystals in the body and decreases the production of inflammatory prostaglandins. Both the stalks and the seeds flush out uric acid crystals, are slightly diuretic and reduce the pain of gout, rheumatoid arthritis and osteoarthritis. Celery also prevents and cures ulcers of the digestive tract since it relaxes the walls of the gut as well as being anti-inflammatory. It is antibacterial, anti-fungal and even discourages some intestinal parasites. Celery reduces cholesterol, triglicerides and LDL (bad fats) and keeps the blood vessels clean and healthy.

How to Use

Above all eat raw, organic celery leaves and stem as often as possible to allay the pain of rheumatoid arthritis, to prevent ulcers and to keep your blood vessels clear of plaque. Eat plenty of celery to keep sperm healthy if you are a man, to prevent menopausal symptoms and PMS is you are a woman. You should consult a trained herbalist for treatment with celery seed for kidney stones, rheumatism, rheumatoid arthritis and osteoarthritis.

Dose
4-8 fresh celery stalks daily.
Celery seed extract tablets or capsules 150-300mg/day.

Contraindications
Avoid celery seed during pregnancy and breastfeeding. People taking thyroxine should not take celery seed, since it inhibits thyroxine uptake. Celery does not cause sensitivity to sunlight by itself but it can cause increased risk of sunburn in people who take prescription ACE inhibitors to control high blood pressure. Many people are allergic to celery so since 2005 the Food Standards Agency has listed it as one of the 12 foods which must be shown clearly on the ingredient list of pre-packed food. Anyone with an allergy to birch pollen, nut or kiwi fruit should not take celery seed.

Chapter 2

Elecampane *Inula helenium*

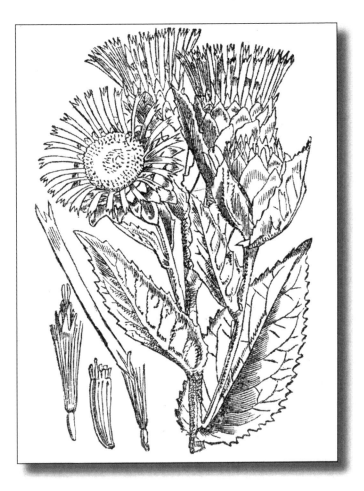

I have been growing elecampane in my garden for several years. It seems quite happy to grow in full sunlight on a south facing slope, as long as I water it regularly. It sends up huge stalks, taller than anything else in my front garden, then in the autumn it produces masses of fluffy seeds which plant themselves in unlikely places, such as between the cracks of the paving in front of my neighbours' houses.

The Romans brought elecampane to Britain and the ancient Celts soon adopted it, giving it a magical status. Some called it Elfwort, for people in ancient times thought that elves caused all sorts of diseases and Elfwort would protect them. It's a magnificent Summer Solstice plant with its golden flowers and giant leaves. Bree Landwalker suggests that elecampane is a powerful herb for banishing and dispelling negative or violent energies, so some pagans sprinkle elecampane powder around their doorways to keep negativity out of their houses. People used to grind the dried herb with vervain and mistletoe to make a love charm powder. In ancient times people believed that fairies loved the yellow flowers and that they could attract love by wearing a sachet of dried flowers round their necks. The Physicians of Myddvai called it the 'Marchalan'. There are many fables about the origin of the Latin name. Gerard tells us: 'It took the name Helenium from Helena, wife of Menelaus, who had her hands full of it when Paris stole her away into Phrygia.' Another legend states that it sprang from her tears: another that Helen first used it against venomous bites; a fourth, that it took the name from the island Helena, where the best plants grew.

The early settlers brought the seeds to North America so that they could use the roots as a horse medicine. Being a member of the Compositae family, it produces hundreds of seeds, which fly away in the wind, so it soon spread across large parts of the continent. It was included in the US Pharmacopeia as a remedy for bronchial congestion.

Botanical Description

Elecampane is one of the tallest members of the Compositae family. It is perennial and grows up to five feet tall, with deeply furrowed, thick stems which branch near the top. The stem and the leaves are downy. At the base of the stalks it produces a rosette of enormous, oval, pointed leaves on long stalks, from one to one and a half feet long and four inches broad in the middle, velvety underneath, with toothed edges. The leaves on the stem become shorter and relatively broader and clasp the stem. It produces very large bright yellow flowers from June to August, three to four inches in diameter, on long stalks. The broad bracts of the leafy involucre under the head are velvety. The root is large and succulent, spindle shaped, branching, brown and aromatic.

Habitat
Damp roadsides and moist fields.

Season
Elecampane flowers in July and August.

How to Grow
Elecampane likes a good, loamy, damp, fairly well-drained soil. Sow the seeds in cold frames or in spring in the open. Propagate elecampane by cutting off pieces of the old root about two inches long, with a bud or eye to each. Plant these nine or ten inches apart in rows about one foot apart. The following spring keep the ground clear of weeds and fork it over in the autumn. The roots will be ready to harvest after two years.

Parts Used
Root and rhizome.

Preservation
Dig up the rhizome and roots of the second- or third-year-old plant in the autumn, scrub clean and dry. Older roots become too woody.

Properties
Elecampane is an aromatic stimulant and tonic. It is also diuretic, diaphoretic, expectorant, antiseptic, astringent and gently stim-

ulant. Herbalists use elecampane for coughs, influenza, bronchitis and asthma. When a person is suffering from bronchitis the lining of the bronchial tubes becomes swollen and red, making it harder to breathe. The inulin in elecampane coats and soothes the lining of the bronchi, acts as an expectorant to make a dry, irritating cough productive and helps to clear congestion from the lungs and bronchi. Since elecampane is bitter it stimulates the flow of bile, the appetite and digestion. The British Herbal Medicine Association states that the sesquiterpene lactones in the roots of elecampane are powerfully antiseptic, healing and relaxant.

Chemical Constituents

In 1804 Rose isolated the polysaccharide, inulin from elecampane root. Several other members of the Compositae, including dahlia roots contain inulin but elecampane is the richest source of it, especially in autumn, when it can contain up to 44%. There is up to 4% volatile oil in elecampane which contains sesquiterpene lactones and several scientists including Bohlmann in 1987 and Huo Yan in 2012, have identified these. They include alantolactone, iso-alantolactone and alantolic acid. Elecampane also contains sterols: beta sitosterol and stigmasterol; triterpenoid saponins, alpha-curcumene; aromadendrene; myristicin. It contains minerals: potassium, calcium, magnesium, iodine, iron, selenium and sodium and vitamins A, C, E, B12, B5, beta-carotene and niacin, resin, pectin and mucilage.

Research

Most of the research on elecampane and its chemical constituents has been carried out in the laboratory. In 1985 Reiter found that elecampane root had a relaxing effect on guinea pig tracheal and ileal smooth muscle. Several scientists, including Bourrel in 1993 and O'Shea in 2009, have demonstrated that elecampane is anti-bacterial. In 1999 Cantrell found that eudesmanolides from the root of elecampane and sweet coneflower (*Rudbeckia subtomentosa*) killed the bacteria that cause tuberculosis (*Mycobacterium tuberculosis*) *in vitro*. The sesquiterpenes in elecampane have many healing effects. In 1999 Cantrell showed that one of the sequiterpene lactones, alantolactone, helps rid the body of intestinal parasites and in 2007 Lim and his team found that several sesquiterpenes from elecampane stimulate detoxifying enzymes to be released in mice. In 2001 Konishi found that seven sesquiterpene lactones in *Inula helenium* roots inhibited cancer cells. In 2015 in Bulgaria Petkova found that elecampane was antioxidant *in vitro*.

In 1977 Luchkova carried out a clinical trial on one hundred and two patients with peptic ulcer disease. He gave them an extract of the eudesmanolides from elecampane. Their symptoms improved. It would be a good idea to carry out a clinical trial with elecampane extract on patients with chronic bronchitis.

How to Use

Make a tincture by chopping up the root and covering it in vodka. Leave for six weeks, before straining it off and storing in a glass container away from the light. Elecampane root is powerful at clearing infections from the lungs. Take 10-15 drops of the tincture several times a day, to treat cough, bronchitis and asthma, but increase the dose and take it as much as 6 times a day if the infection is acute. Only take elecampane to treat an active infection. It will help relax the trachea and bronchi, make a dry cough productive and soothe the throat. Combine elecampane root decoction or tincture with mullein to make a cough mixture or take a cough syrup or lozenges containing elecampane. Also use to aid digestion, to relieve night sweats and to lift your spirits.

Dose

2-3 mls of tincture.

1-2 grams dried root as a tea or in capsule form.

Contraindications

Elecampane is generally safe and well-tolerated as long as it is used in moderation, especially for the young or elderly. Excessive doses will upset the stomach. Do not take during pregnancy or breastfeeding. People with diabetes or heart problems should not take elecampane. Large doses can cause diarrhoea and vomiting. People who are allergic to Asteraceae family pollen (chrysanthemum, chamomile, ragweed, daisy) may be allergic to elecampane.

Chapter 3

Garlic *Allium sativum*

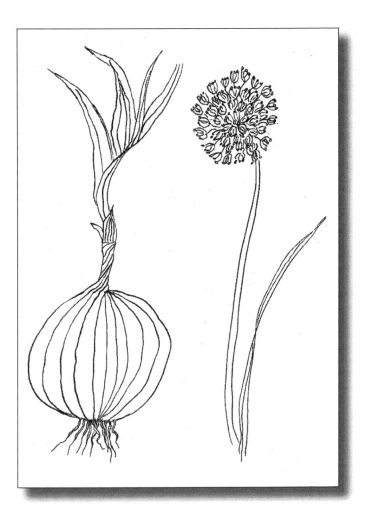

I remember my sister-in-law telling me how when she was a child, living in north Italy, she had to drink milk with garlic cooked in it, to expel a tapeworm. She described pulling the whole tapeworm out. It was incredibly long. I don't know which was more disgusting – the description of the tapeworm or the description of the cure! Years later, when I was breastfeeding my babies my nipples bled. A naturopath prescribed an ointment made from lanolin and garlic, which healed my nipples. So my babies consumed small quantities of garlic at a very young age!

Garlic originated somewhere between West China, Kazakhstan and Kyrgyzstan. Archaeologists in Egypt have discovered 3700 BCE sculptures of garlic bulbs. The Egyptians fed garlic to their slaves so that they would not need so much food but would be strong and work harder. Herodotus wrote: 'Inscriptions on the plates of the Egyptian pyramids tell us how much their builders used the garlic for this vegetable, 1600 talents of silver were spent' (approximately 30 million dollars). The Egyptian Ebers papyrus (around 1500 BCE) mentions various medicinal plants, including garlic, which it says can be used to heal thirty-two illnesses. Archaeologists found garlic bulbs in the pyramids and in Tutankhamen's tomb. The Chinese and the Sumerians were using garlic as a medicine from 2700 BCE. Indian priests were the first physicians in ancient India and they used garlic as a tonic, together with spells, rituals, prayers and secret ceremonies. The ancient Indian Vedas mention garlic.

It was grown in the gardens of Babylon, and the local population used to call it a 'rank rose'. Ashurbanipal, the last great tsar of Assyria, hid ten thousand volumes of clay plates which recorded the life, customs and rituals of the Babylonian-Assyrian world, including volumes devoted to medicinal plants. The first Assyrian book of medicinal plants describes how physicians used garlic to bring down body temperature, as a remedy against constipation and muscle inflammation and to kill intestinal parasites.

From Egypt garlic spread round the shores of the Mediterranean to Palestine, Greece and ancient Rome. Archeologists excavating Knossos Palace on Crete found garlic bulbs dating from 1850-1400 BCE. Early Greek army leaders fed their army with garlic before major battles. According to Theophrastus (370-285

BCE), the Greeks offered garlic bulbs to their Gods. Hippocrates (459-370 BCE) wrote that garlic would kill intestinal parasites. Dioscorides (40-90 CE) recommended garlic for colic relief, to kill intestinal parasites, for regulating the menstrual cycle and against seasickness. In the Middle Ages, people in Europe used garlic to prevent them from catching the plague. In 1720 four thieves in Marseilles were offered freedom in exchange for them burying the plague dead. They made a mixture of chopped garlic and wine, which they drank all day while burying the dead and survived the plague.

The ancient Romans used garlic as a remedy and a food and when they invaded Britain they brought garlic with them. The ancient Celts soon learned to use garlic as a medicine, though it would be a long time before they began to use it as a food. Indeed many people in Britain still do not eat garlic today.

Botanical Description

Garlic is a member of the lily family or Liliaceae with long, smooth, flat leaves eight millimetres wide. The greenish, whitish flowers are at the end of a stalk rising straight up from the bulb, grouped together in a globular head, or umbel, with an enclosing leaf, and among them are small bulbils. Garlic has a compound bulb, consisting of numerous cloves, which fit together between membraneous scales, enclosed within a whitish skin.

Season

Garlic is ready to harvest in the spring and if you leave it in the ground it will flower in the summer.

Cultivation

Dig plenty of compost and/or well rotted manure into the soil and plant your garlic bulbs in early spring.

Garlic *Allium sativum*

Parts Used
The bulb.

Preservation
Garlic will keep for a long time if you store it in a cool place.

Properties
Garlic contains sulphur glycosides, which give it its character-istic smell. Garlic is powerfully antibacterial, antiviral, antiox-idant and anti-parasitic. It protects from LDL cholesterol (bad fats). It decreases the concentration of triglycerides and choles-terol in blood and prevents them from sticking to the sides of the blood vessels, so reducing the risk of atherosclerosis and heart diseases. Since humans excrete allicin partly through the lungs herbalists use garlic to treat respiratory tract diseases.

Chemical Constituents
Scientists began investigating the chemical content of garlic in 1844. By 1892 they had isolated several aliphatic unsaturat-ed sulphur compounds, but it was not until 1944 that Cavallito and Bailey identified allicin, a tricky job because it is extremely unstable. In 1947 scientists worked out the chemical formula of allicin and discovered that alliin which is not antibacterial, is converted to allicin by alliinase. Allicin, the major active com-pound in garlic, is powerfully antibacterial, but quickly con-verts to ajoene. Garlic contains many other sulphur containing compounds, such as allyl disulphide, and allyl trisulphide, etc. In 2000 Superko isolated six powerful phenylpropanoids from garlic peel. It contains quercetin, cellulose, amino acids, lip-ids, etheric oil, complex of fructosans (carbohydrates), steroid saponosides, organic acids, vitamins (C, A, and B complex), en-zymes etc. It contains minerals: manganese, potassium, calcium, phosphorous, magnesium, selenium, germanium, sodium, iron, zinc and copper.

Research

In 2007 Tedeschi and his team carried out *in vitro* studies on garlic which showed that it was antibiotic, antibacterial and antifungal. Recent studies have revealed that garlic protects from the common cold. Several scientists, including Agarwal in 1996, Sovová in 2004 and Kovacevic in 2000, have demonstrated that garlic and compounds isolated from garlic, including allicin, lower cholesterol and blood pressure *in vivo*. Several scientists, including Amagase in 2001, have demonstrated *in vivo* and *in vitro* that ajoenes from garlic prevent thrombosis. Garlic prevents free radicals from forming and helps the body to destroy them. In 2001 and 2006 Borek carried out research on patients suffering from diseases that affect the heart and blood vessels of the body and the brain, including Alzheimer's disease. Since garlic is antioxidant, lowers cholesterol, prevents blood clots and lowers blood pressure it may help to prevent dementia.

Agarwal mentions that garlic extract stops cancer cells from dividing and multiplying in all phases, without unwanted side effects. In 2004 Hassan demonstrated *in vivo* that ajoene is powerfully active against leukaemia. Scientists from Britain believe that high doses of garlic extract can help prevent cancer.

In 2008 Ried and his team in Australia reviewed and analysed all the trials that had been carried out to investigate the effect of garlic on blood pressure. Altogether 252 people took the garlic powder and 251 people were in the control group. When they analysed the 10 studies involving people with high systolic blood pressure they found that the people taking the garlic improved significantly. Their systolic blood pressure went down by an average of 4.56 mm Hg. People with normal systolic blood pressure remained unchanged by the garlic. People with high diastolic blood pressure who took the garlic powder also improved significantly. Their diastolic blood pressure went down by an average of 7.27 mm Hg. Again people with normal diastolic blood pressure were not affected by the garlic powder.

In 2015 Rohner and his team also reviewed and analysed nine trials which demonstrated that garlic brings down high blood pressure. They found that systolic and diastolic blood pressure went down in the patients who took the garlic compared to the controls. Interestingly they found that some garlic preparations were more effective at reducing high blood pressure than others. This is because different preparations contain different chemical constituents. For example, one product may contain more oil-soluble compounds and another may contain more water-soluble compounds. A few of the patients suffered bloating, flatulence and reflux as a result of taking the garlic. More research is needed to understand how garlic lowers blood pressure, especially in the long term and which garlic preparations are the most effective.

Today, many pharmacopoeias throughout the world, including the European Pharmacopoeia, the United States pharmacopoeia and the British Pharmacopoeia, prescribe garlic as well as garlic preparations.

How to Use

The German Commission E recommends that people with high levels of cholesterol should eat fresh garlic or take it as a supplement to prevent hardening of the arteries. If you tolerate garlic you can eat large amounts of it and indeed many people, especially in southern Europe, do. People who suffer from gastric diseases and people who produce too much hydrochloric acid cannot tolerate garlic. Therefore many manufacturers produce garlic capsules, to stimulate appetite and nervous system, to lower high cholesterol and high blood pressure, to prevent arteriosclerosis, to kill children's parasites, as antiseptic and so on. Not all of these preparations are effective. If possible raw garlic is the best remedy. Eating raw garlic every day will prevent colds and influenza, keep the blood vessels supple and healthy, keep the brain functioning and prevent dementia in old age. It will dissolve blood clots that sometimes form as a result of bruising.

Dose

Four grams of fresh garlic or garlic capsules per day.

Contraindications

Some people suffer a burning sensation in the mouth and intestine, nausea, sickness and odour from the breath and the body. Some people find it causes problems when applied to their skin. Garlic may interfere with some prescribed medicines.

Chapter 4

Lavender *Lavandula angustifolia*

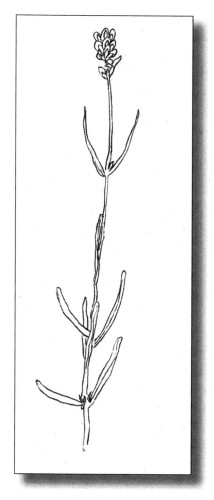

When I was a child my mother used to cut the long lavender stalks when the bush produced its purple flowers and bring the fragrant pile into the kitchen. I would run each stalk through a fork to pull the flowers off into a bowl. She gave me pieces of patterned cloth to sew into little bags, which I stuffed with the tiny purple flowers, then stitched up. We put these little sachets among our clothes to keep the moths at bay and make our clothes smell sweet. We didn't dry our lavender before we sewed it into bags but let the moisture gradually evaporate through the material. It didn't seem to make our clothes damp, but then it was summer and the sun shone through the windows.

Lavender is an aromatic shrub native to the Mediterranean hills, much loved by the Romans, who brought it to Britain when they invaded. The word lavender comes from the Latin *lavare*, meaning to wash, for the Romans added it to their baths. When lavender grows in the hot southern Mediterranean countries, each kilo of the dried flowers produces at least thirteen millilitres of essential oil. It grows well in Britain but it does not produce the same quantities of essential oil. People have been growing lavender for centuries and extracting the essential oil by steam distillation or water distillation. People have long known that it relieves anxiety and depression. According to Blumenthal people used lavender to disinfect hospitals and sick rooms in ancient Persia, Greece and Rome.

Botanical Description

Lavender grows as a bush, between one and three feet high, with a short, irregular, crooked, much-branched stem, covered with greyish bark which flakes off. It has numerous straight broom-like, bluntly-quadrangular branches, covered in fine hairs. The leaves grow opposite each other, attached to the stem directly, without stalks. When they are young the leaves are white with dense hairs on both sides. When they are full grown, they are green, one and a half inches long with scattered hairs above and finely downy underneath. Lavender produces flowers in blunt spikes on long stems. The spikes consist of whorls or rings of between six and ten flowers with very short stalks. The flowers are tubular and ribbed, with thirteen veins, purple-grey, five-toothed and hairy.

Habitat

Lavender is native to a number of countries from Cape Verde and the Canary Islands to northern Africa and from southern Spain to south east India but it seems to grow best in the southern Mediterranean countries of Spain, Italy and France.

Season

Lavender flowers in May, June and July.

How to Grow

Lavender likes a dry, open, well drained, sunny position and a poor or moderately fertile, chalky or alkaline soil. On heavier soils such as clay or clay loam, lavender doesn't live very long. If your soil is heavy add organic matter and gravel to improve the drainage and plant on a mound. It doesn't like frost, strong winds or being waterlogged. However, it will grow well in Britain, especially on a south facing slope. Clear the weeds from land where you want to plant the lavender in the autumn. Then dig in some well rotted manure and leave to lie fallow until the following spring, when you should dig up any remaining weeds and dig the whole area. You can grow lavender from seed sown in April, but people usually propagate it from cuttings or by dividing the roots. Take cuttings in August and September, pot them up and plant them out in the following spring. Don't let the young plants flower during the first year, so that they become nice and bushy.

You can grow lavender in large pots, 30-40 cm diameter, using a loam-based compost with extra coarse grit, up to 30% by volume to improve the drainage. Water the pots well in the summer but keep them fairly dry in the winter by standing them in a greenhouse or in the rain shadow of a wall. Lavender really doesn't like getting its roots soaking wet too often. After all in its native country it doesn't rain nearly as much as it does in Britain, and lavender usually grows in poor soil that the water drains off quickly.

Prune your lavender every year to keep it compact. Cut the flower stalks off and remove about 2.5 cm (one inch) of the current year's growth in the late summer.

Parts Used

The flowers and leaves.

Preservation

Cut the stems when they are flowering, in the morning after the dew has evaporated and the plant is dry but before the sun gets too hot. Hang the lavender stems upside down in a well ventilated place, out of the sun, to dry.

Properties

Lavender, is anti-depressive, diuretic, anti-inflammatory, anti-bacterial, expectorant and anti-fungal. Since it is anti-spasmodic, stimulates the flow or bile, stops gas forming in the digestive system and calms the stomach, it helps to promote healthy digestion. It is effective for burns and insect bites. It is mildly sedative, hypnotic and anti-convulsant. It is analgesic, so relieves the pain of rheumatism and arthritis. It stimulates the hair to grow. Lavender works on the physical as well as the psycho-spiritual planes and people have long known that it relieves anxiety and depression and improves mood.

Dr Otto Warburg, twice Nobel laureate for his cancer research, discovered that human cells have an electric charge and Bruce Tanio, head of the Department of Agriculture at Washington University measured the frequency of this charge. He found that negative thoughts diminish our frequency and positive thoughts raise it. Robert O Becker, doctor and author of *The Body Electric*, says that a person's health can be determined by measuring this frequency. Bruce Tanio also measured the frequencies of essential oils and their effect on human cell frequencies when they are applied to the body. He found that certain essential oils can raise the body's frequency. This could partly explain how lavender essential oil improves mood and relieves anxiety and depression.

Chemical Constituents

Lavandula angustifolia contains essential oil, composed up at least thirty-eight different compounds: monoterpenes including alpha-pinene, camphor, limonene; monoterpene alcohols, including borneol, linalool (which is sedative, local anaesthetic and anti-bacterial); monoterpene aldehydes: cumin aldehyde; monoterpene ethers, including cineole (which is antifungal and antispasmodic), monoterpene esters, including linalyl acetate (which is sedative, local anaesthetic and anti-bacterial); monoterpene ketones, including carvone and coumarin (which is anti-inflammatory); benzenoids, including eugenol (which is anti-spasmodic, local anaesthetic and anti-bacterial), rosmarinic acid (which is anti-bacterial), thymol; and sesquiterpenes, including alpha-santal.

The proportions of these compounds varies according to the time of the year and the place where the lavender grows. These compounds are also present in different proportions in different species of lavender.

Research

In 1910 Rene-Maurice Gattefosse, a chemist who made perfumes, was severely burned on both hands. In his book *Aromatherapy*, he wrote that he put his hands into a basin full of cold water with lavender essential oil in it and this prevented blisters forming. He was so impressed by the powerful effect of lavender essential oil that he began using and studying its effects on burned soldiers in military hospitals during World War One. Since then there has been masses of research into the medicinal properties of all the different species of lavender, much of it carried out in the laboratory. It would not be appropriate for me to cover all

of this research since I'm not writing a book solely about lavender, so I've picked out a few of the properties of this miraculous
plant that have been proven, along with a few of the properties
of some of the different compounds in it.

In 1992 Jager found that up to ninety per cent of *Lavandula angustifolia* essential oil was composed of two compounds: linalyl
acetate and linalool (which are sedative, anaesthetic, antibacterial, anti-fungal and insecticidal). When he applied the essential
oil (diluted in a vegetable oil) to the skin of volunteers, the two
compounds absorbed through the skin into the blood stream in
five minutes, had been completely absorbed in nineteen minutes
and remained in the bloodstream for up to one and a half hours.
So during a whole body massage with lavender essential oil, the
oil travels through the skin into the blood stream, which carries
it round the body until it reaches the lungs, the kidneys and liver, where it leaves the body. It probably reaches all the organs,
including the brain, on its journey round the body, possibly even
all the cells in the body, since it is fat soluble and passes through
membranes. Scientists have detected linalyl acetate and linalool
on people's breath when they were being massaged with lavender essential oil. These compounds also absorb into the blood
when the patient breathes in lavender oil vapour.

Many essential oils, including lavender, are anti-bacterial.
There has been an enormous amount of research into the anti-bacterial properties of lavender, including that by Roller in
2009 who demonstrated that the essential oils of several different lavender species inhibited drug resistant bacteria at very low
concentrations. There are many anti-bacterial compounds in lavender, including eugenol, rosmarinic acid, alpha-terpineol and
camphor. Rosmarinic acid is also anti-oxidant.

Various different species of lavender are anti-fungal, as demonstrated by various scientists, including Dauria in 2005 and Zuzarte
in 2011, who both demonstrated that the essential oil from *Lavandula viridis* and *Lavandula angustifolia* killed many different species

of fungi, including *Candida albicans* at low concentrations. *Candida albicans* can cause thrush if it grows out of control, especially in the vagina, resulting in itching and irritation. Lavender species contain many different anti-fungal compounds, including alpha-pinene, cineole, beta-pinene and p-cymene. In 2002 Cassella investigated the antifungal activity of *Lavandula angustifolia* and tea tree (*Melaleuca alternifolia*) essential oil, used together to treat tinea. Tinea is the name of a group of diseases caused by fungi. They include ringworm, athlete's foot and jock itch. Cassella showed that the combination of the two essential oils was more powerful than the individual essential oils used separately. He used it to kill two species of funghi that cause tinea.

In 2006 Moon and her team tested essential oils of *Lavandula angustifolia* and *Lavandula intermedia* against *Giardia duodenalis* and *Trichomonas vaginalis*. *Giardia duodenalis* is a very common human parasite which infects the intestines and causes diarrhoea, bloating, gas and stomach pain. *Trichomonas vaginalis* is a common human parasite that is usually sexually transmitted. She demonstrated that very low concentrations of the essential oils (less than one per cent) completely killed the parasites. This suggests that you could use a solution of lavender tincture or essential oil in water as a douche to treat *Trichomonas vaginalis*. But it is difficult to say whether lavender oil taken internally would work to cure *Giardia duodenalis*. In 1999 Ghelardini and team demonstrated the anaesthetic action of *Lavandula angustifolia* on rabbits. Many different scientists have demonstrated the sedative effects of *Lavandula angustifolia*, including Buchbauer in 1991 and Guillemain in 1989. Several scientists have demonstrated the anti-spasmodic effect of lavender, including Lis-Balchin in 1997 and in 1999.

The lavender plant converts limonene into perillyl alcohol. There is some perillyl alcohol in *L angustifolia* but *Lavandula latifolia* has a lot more of it. In 1999 Zhang and team found that perillyl alcohol protected against cancers forming *in vitro*. Pharmaceutical companies are busy investigating perillyl alcohol, carrying out clinical trials against breast cancer with it.

Manufacturers sometimes obtain lavender essential oil by steam distillation, pumping steam through the lavender flowers in a large metal vessel. The steam removes the essential oil and leaves the vessel through a pipe to a water-cooled condenser. The steam and the volatile oil both re-condense and drip into a glass flask where they separate into two layers, the volatile oil forming the top layer. The aqueous solution (the condensed steam) contains small amounts of essential oil and the water soluble compounds from the plant. This is called a hydrosol or hydrolat. There is no need to dilute lavender hydrolat/hydrosol, which can be used directly on the skin. In China there are more than two hundred manufacturers making hydrosols from nearly thirty different plants including rose and chamomile. Several different scientists, including Kunicka-Styczynska in 2015 have suggested that the antibacterial and anti-fungal properties of *Lavandula angustifolia* hydrosol makes it an ideal preservative for cosmetics such as moisturisers. In 2014 DeHart and Whalen documented that lavender hydrosol together with lavender essential oil is effective for treating minor burns. They demonstrated that by using lavender you can prevent blisters from forming after a first degree burn. In 2016 Lee covered the closed eyes of twenty students suffering from long term stress with cotton sheets moistened with lavender hydrosol. Their heart rates returned to normal and their stress levels reduced.

Several different scientists, including Woelk in 2010, have demonstrated that lavender relieves anxiety. Woelk found that silexan, a new lavender oil capsule, worked as well as lorazepam at reducing anxiety in a clinical trial, without causing sleepiness or being addictive, (the side effects of lorazepam). In 2004 Basch demonstrated in another clinical trial that lavender hydrolat relieves anxiety and depression and promotes sleep. Also in 2004 Park and Lee gave nursing students lavender vapour to reduce stress. The nursing students reported that they felt less anxious and the physical symptoms of anxiety were reduced. Several scientists, including Lewith in 2005, have demonstrated that *Lavandula angustifolia* inhalations help insomniacs to sleep.

Many different scientists, including Louis and Kowalski in 2002 have demonstrated that lavender aromatherapy decreases pain, anxiety and depression in hospice patients. It also promotes an increased sense of well-being. Also in 2002 Morris carried out two trials with lavender baths to promote psychological well-being. He found that it reduced anger, frustration and negative thoughts about the future. A number of different scientists, including Akhondzadeh in 2003, have demonstrated that lavender can help people suffering from depression. Akhondzadeh and team carried out a clinical trial to compare *L angustifolia* tincture with imipramine, to treat mild to moderate depression. They found that *Lavandula* on its own was less effective than imipramine but the combination of imipramine and *Lavandula* tincture was more effective than imipramine on its own.

Several scientists, including Hur in 2004, have demonstrated that lavender oil helps cuts to heal. In 2004 Hur and Han carried out a clinical trial on women who had been given episiotomy during the birth of their babies. They found that lavender oil helped the cut to heal and prevented bacterial infection. The anti-inflammatory compounds, coumarin and caryophyllene in *Lavandula angustifolia* soothed the healing cut, while the many anti-bacterial compounds kept it clean. Other compounds promoted healing.

In 1997 Charron made 40 adults with blocked sinuses inhale the essential oil of *L latifolia*. The patients said that they felt their sinuses clearing and they began to cough up mucus while they were inhaling. This lasted between twenty minutes and two hours after the inhalation and all the patients said they felt better after the treatment.

Several scientists, including Lis-Balchin in 1999, have demonstrated that lavender oil has an antispasmodic effect on smooth muscle. This effect is due to the compounds linalyl acetate and linalool, present in lavender. The human intestines are lined with smooth muscle, so although the scientists carried out their experiments on the smooth muscle from rats and guinea pigs, which is different from the smooth muscle in humans, there is a possibility that lavender essential oil is antispasmodic in humans. This would explain the soothing effect lavender has on indigestion and upset stomach.

In 1999 Yurkova demonstrated that lavender aromatherapy helped men to recover from exercise. At the end of the rest period the blood pressure of the lavender-treated group was lower, and their hearts were beating slower, compared with the control group.

Many different scientists, including Smith in 2003, and Lin in 2007 have demonstrated that lavender essential oil inhalations calm elderly dementia patients and help them to recover a little of their memory.

How to Use

Make a tea out of dried lavender for restlessness, palpitations, insomnia, upset stomach, indigestion, mild headache and laryngitis. Make an infusion of dried lavender and use as a douche to treat candida infections.

Use lavender essential oil diluted in vegetable oil and massage to relieve muscle pain. Rub into sunburn to take the redness out of it. Diluted lavender oil will even prevent scar tissue from forming and reduce scars that have already formed. Massage your lower abdomen with diluted oil to ease painful periods. Massage into the temples to relieve a headache. Use it to treat insect bites, burns, inflammation, itching and for healing small cuts. Use it to treat eczema in small children.

Breathe in the vapour of lavender essential oil throughout the day, or put a drop on each wrist to bring down high blood pressure and calm palpitations. Breathe in the vapour to help you sleep, to improve your mood and raise your spirits. Add the essential oil to boiling water in a bowl and inhale the steam with a towel over your head to calm an asthma attack, to help clear up bronchitis, pharyngitis, sinusitis and laryngitis. Put two drops of pure essential oil behind your children's ears (never inside the ears) to cure earache. Comb lavender oil into your children's hair to prevent them from catching lice. Add a few drops of lavender oil to your bath to help you relax. Mix lavender and tea tree essential oils and rub between your toes to cure athlete's foot.

Make a lavender hydrosol by heating lavender flowers in distilled water in a large saucepan in which you have placed a trivet. The trivet should be well above the level of the water. Put a bowl on the trivet and put the saucepan lid on upside down. Fill the saucepan lid with ice. You will have to keep replacing the ice as it melts. The steam will rise from the saucepan, hit the cold lid, condense and drip back into the bowl. This is your hydrolat. Store it in the fridge in a glass jar and use it to clean cuts and scrapes, to cool a burn, to remove makeup, to relieve pain and relax the body and mind. If refrigerated it will keep for a few weeks. Lavender hydrolat will help to heal the burns caused by radiation therapy.

Dose

Essential Oil

6 drops added to a 20 litre bath.

2-4 drops in 720 ml boiling water for inhalation.

1 ml lavender essential oil in 10 mls of vegetable oil for a massage oil.

1-4 drops can be taken internally.

Lavender Herb

1-2 teaspoons lavender steeped in a cup of boiling water.

Contraindications

Lavender essential oil is safe, as long as you dilute it in a vegetable oil, though a few people are allergic to it. Do not use it during the first three months of pregnancy or on babies before they are six months old. Lavender may increase the risk of bleeding if you give it to people who are taking anticoagulants. Lavender may increase the narcotic and sedative effects of anti-convulsants. Do not take large doses of lavender orally since it can cause nausea, vomiting and anorexia. There are a multitude of different varieties of lavender with different properties. To be on the safe side stick to *Lavandula angustifolia*. There are an awful lot of poor quality essential oils on the market, diluted with alcohol and other additives. Only one hundred per cent pure essential oils really work.

Chapter 5

Marigold *Calendula officinalis*

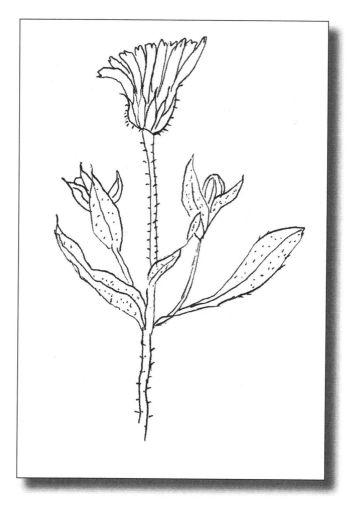

Calendula flowers continuously for months on end in my allot-ment, scattering its seeds around itself if I don't pick the flowers in time. Every year I collect hundreds of flowers and lay them out on my dining table, occupying three quarters of the table while they dry, when I pick the petals off and press them into a glass jar with sunflower oil to macerate in the sun.

The Romans brought *Calendula* seed with them when they invaded Britain, but the ancient Celts living along the south coast of Britain may well have been growing the flowers long before that. Marigold grows easily in Britain, making a beautiful display with its bright flowers. The name *Calendula* comes from the Latin Kalendae for 'first day of the month' because you can find it blooming almost every month of the year in Italy. In England winter is a much longer affair than in Southern Europe so it only blooms for half the year. The Physicians of Myddvai made marigold ointments by boiling the flowers with butter, rosin, suet and wax, then straining it under a press. Historically people used to use it as a substitute saffron, to colour and flavour foods such as butter, cheese, custard, bread, biscuits, soups and rice dishes. People also added the petals to salads and used it as a dye for fabric and hair. The pharmaceutical industry uses the bright orange pigment to colour some medicines.

Botanical Description

Marigold is a small, bushy, annual plant, thirty to fifty centimetres high with light green, lance-shaped hairy leaves which grow out of alternate sides of the stem. Each stem has a flower at its tip up to 3 inches in diameter and is erect, angular, downy and branched. Each flower has an epicalyx of numerous narrow, pointed green sepals, densely covered with glandular hairs and orange male petals radiating out from the centre. Female ray florets, that look like orange petals, are arranged round them.

Habitat

Calendula is native to the Southern Mediterranean, North Africa and western Asia. It grows in gardens, waste lands, roadsides and near villages from 0-1000 metres altitude.

Season

Calendula flowers from spring right through to early November in Britain. In the Mediterranean it flowers almost all year round at low altitudes.

How to Grow

Calendula is very easy to grow from seed. Simply scatter the seeds on well dug soil.

Parts Used

Flowers and leaves.

Preservation

Lay the flowers out flat to dry in a warm, airy place, away from the sun. Or if you want to dry the whole plant, hang the stalks up to dry.

Properties

The flowers reduce fever, are astringent, anti-spasmodic, anti-inflammatory, antimicrobial, antibacterial, anti-fungal, anti-tumour, anti-HIV and wound healing. Marigold helps regulate the female menstrual cycle. The seed has antioxidant properties. The flowers accelerate bacterial degradation of organic material so if you grow too many of them add them to your compost to speed it up.

Chemical Constituents

A great many scientists have isolated and identified the many compounds in *Calendula officinalis* flowers, leaves and roots. In 2009 Muley reviewed the work that had been carried out so far.

Calendula flowers contain a wonderful array of compounds with healing properties: terpenoids, including sitosterols, stigmasterols and saponins; all sorts of flavonoids, including quercetin, rutin, calendoflaside; coumarins, including scopoletin, umbelliferone and esculetin. They contain saponins and qui-

nones, including alpha-tocopherol (vitamin E.) They contain up
to 0.4% volatile oil which is composed of a great number of compounds including monoterpenes, triterpenes, for example: calenduloside and sesquiterpenes, such as alpha pinene, limonene
and geraniol. The wonderful colour comes from carotenoids,
including neoxanthin, lutein, alpha carotene. There are fifteen
amino acids in the flowers, together with lipids, including linoleic and linolenic acids. They contain polysaccharides, which
stimulate the immune system. Whole *Calendula* flowers also contain oleoresins, which can be extracted using 90% ethanol and
10% water mixture.

Research

There has been an enormous amount of research into the healing
properties of *Calendula* flowers, as well as the individual compounds in them, and again it would not be appropriate for me
to cover it all. Much of the research focusses on the wound healing properties of *Calendula*. In 2008 Leach reviewed the evidence
that the flowers heal wounds and Chandran demonstrated this
in the laboratory. In order for wounds to heal the body needs
to grow new blood vessels around the wound, to transport all
the nutrients needed to make new cells. In 1996 Patrick and his
team demonstrated *in vitro* that an aqueous extract of the flowers stimulated capillaries to grow. During the second phase in
wound healing new cells need to grow, to replace those that
were destroyed. In 1982 Klouchek-Popova demonstrated that
Calendula flower extract ointment stimulated the cells around a
wound to grow in rats. In 2008 Preethi gave *Calendula* flower
extract to rats to drink. It speeded up the healing process on
their burns. Many of the flavonoids in *Calendula* flowers are antioxidant and wound healing and several scientists, including
Popovic in 1999 and Frankic in 2008, have demonstrated the antioxidant properties. Frankic found that the petals were the most
strongly antioxidant. In 2002 Cordova found that a *Calendula*

flower extract which was full of flavonoids and terpenoids acted as a free radical scavenger, was antioxidant and protected liver microsomes from damage. In 1994 Loggia found that *Calendula* flower ointment relieved sore nipple pain. In 2005 Duran treated varicose vein ulcers successfully using *Calendula* ointment.

Inflammation is a symptom of many different conditions, including rheumatism, rheumatoid arthritis, bruising, burns, sore throats, bronchitis etc. Even wounds can become inflamed. Some of the terpenoids in *Calendula* are anti-inflammatory. Several scientists, including Della in 1994 and Ukiya in 2006 have demonstrated that a *Calendula* flower extract is anti-inflammatory and that triterpenoids are responsible for this effect. In 2005 Fuchs demonstrated that a *Calendula*/rosemary cream protected the skin from irritant contact dermatitis caused by letting the skin come into contact with sodium laurel sulfate (found in soaps, shampoos, toothpaste and detergents). Swelling is another common symptom that can be caused by inflammation, bruising, sprains etc. In 1997 Zitteri-Eglseer and team demonstrated that the main triterpendiol esters of *Calendula officinalis* flowers reduced oedema (swelling) in mice.

Calendula flower extract is anti-bacterial, anti-viral and highly anti-fungal. Many scientists including Iauk in 2003 have demonstrated the anti-bacterial properties of the flower extracts against a range of bacteria. Several scientists, including Gazim in 2008 have demonstrated that the extracts are anti-fungal against various fungi, including *Candida* species. In 1997 Kalvatene and his team showed that extracts of *Calendula officinalis* flowers were anti-viral against HIV *in vitro* and in 1970 Bogdanova demonstrated the anti-viral effect of *Calendula* tincture against influenza and herpes viruses.

Several terpenoids are anti-tumour and in 2006 Ukiya and his team isolated an anti-cancer compound: calenduloside from *Calendula officinalis* flowers, which was active against various different cancer cells. Also in 2006 Medina and his team found that

Calendula officinalis flower extracts inhibited several different kinds of cancer cells. They also found that the extracts activated immune system cells, including natural killer cells: white blood cells which destroy cancer cells in our bodies. In 1989 Varlijen found that polysaccharides from *Calendula officinalis* stimulated immune cells.

In 2006 Bashir demonstrated in the laboratory that extracts of *Calendula officinalis* flowers relaxed the walls of the intestine. In 2007 Alexenizor demonstrated that extracts of the flowers were insecticidal.

In 2004 In France Pommier carried out a randomised clinical trial to compare *Calendula officinalis* with trolamine for preventing acute dermatitis during irradiation after breast cancer surgery. He chose 254 women aged between 18 and 75 years, who had been operated on for breast cancer and were now receiving radiation therapy. He gave half of them *Calendula* ointment (Pommade au Calendula par Digestion, by Boiron Ltd, Levallois-Perret, France) and the other half trolamine ointment. The women who used the *Calendula* ointment experienced significantly less pain than the women who used the trolamine ointment, and none of the *calendula* group had any allergic reactions. Four of the women using the trolamine ointment had allergic reactions. This clinical trial suggests that women who have had radiation therapy after breast cancer surgery can safely use *calendula* ointment to prevent dermatitis. In 2002 Barnes found that *calendula* ointment reduced the pain that can occur when mastectomy causes lymphedema. The anti-inflammatory and anti-swelling compounds in *calendula* probably help the lymphedema.

In 1992 Lievre carried out a randomised, parallel group study with 156 patients with second and third degree burns. They compared *calendula* ointment with Elase (a proteolytic ointment; Pfizer, New York, NY) and petroleum jelly. The *calendula* ointment was better tolerated than petroleum jelly alone for healing.

How to Use

Marigold flowers and young leaves are edible. Add them to salads. Use the petals to colour and flavour soups, cakes and creamed vegetables.

Calendula is one of the best wound healing herbs. It prevents infection of severe wounds, reduces inflammation and increases circulation in the skin, which speeds up the healing process. Use *calendula* tincture and ointment to heal bruises, burns, cuts and minor infections. It is particularly good for injured, irritated, sensitive and inflamed skin. Make a wash to treat cuts by pouring one cupful of boiling water over a spoonful of dried petals. Leave to steep for ten minutes and use for skin and mucous membrane inflammations, such as pharyngitis, leg ulcers, boils, bed sores, gum inflammation and rashes. You can also use lotions, poultices and compresses made with *calendula* flowers. Sit in a bath full of *calendula* flowers (dried or fresh) after giving birth, to soothe and heal and prevent bacterial infection. Make an infusion from the whole flowers and take to treat colds, coughs and flu, as well as acne, spots, boils and yeast infections. It will stimulate the immune system to eliminate bacteria and viruses, the liver to break down toxins and stimulate the lymphatic system to increase lymphatic drainage, which rids the body of toxins.

The German Commission E has approved the use of *calendula* flower internally and topically for inflammation of the mucous membranes of the mouth and throat, and externally for poorly healing wounds and foot ulcers. Take *calendula* tincture or infusion of the flowers to treat stomach ulcers and liver complaints. Make a *calendula* flower tea to cleanse the blood and treat eczema, boils and adolescent acne.

Make *calendula* oil by drying the flowers, then removing the petals, putting them into a glass jar, covering them in vegetable oil and leaving them in the sunshine until the oil turns bright orange. Strain the oil from the petals and store it in a glass bottle.

You can also make a *calendula* flower oil using the whole flowers. This will contain the waxes and resins from the sepals. To make an ointment, heat the oil and add grated beeswax, a spoonful at the time. Test the firmness of the ointment by dropping a drop on a china plate. If it is too soft add more beeswax. If it is too hard, add more infused oil. Use the ointment for inflamed nipples, burns, bruises and sunburn. Make hypercal ointment by adding *hypericum* flower oil to the *calendula* oil before adding the melted beeswax. Hypericum is another plant with remarkable healing qualities which works well together with *calendula*. There is a chapter on Hypericum in my book *The Healing Power of Celtic Plants*.

Dose

25-75 drops of tincture 1-4 times a day.

Make an infusion with one ounce of the flowers in one pint of boiling water.

Contraindications

Pregnant women should not take *calendula* internally because it can stimulate menstrual activity. People who are allergic to the plant family Asteraceae may be allergic to *calendula*.

Chapter 6

Rosemary *Rosmarinus officinalis*

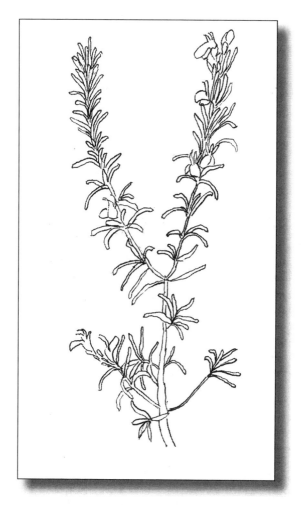

The Romans brought rosemary to Britain and by the thirteenth century the Physicians of Myddvai were using it to cure head-aches and other symptoms. The ancient Celts were almost cer-tainly using it medicinally after the Roman invasion, at least in the south of the country, where they may well have started growing it before that. Rosemary is one of the few plants that has been used for many centuries at both weddings and funerals. Hamlet said to Ophelia: 'There's rosemary, that's for remembrance,' reminding us that already in Shakespeare's time rosemary had a reputation for aiding memory.

Botanical Description

Rosemary belongs to the mint family, the Lamiaceae, and is related to basil, thyme, mint and sage. It is an evergreen perennial shrub, with strongly aromatic, needle-like evergreen leaves ten to forty millimetres long and two to four millemetres wide with recurved edges. The upper surface of the leaves is dark green and shiny, the lower surface is greyish-green and densely hairy with a prominent midrib. The flowers are purplish white and two-lipped with two protruding stamens.

Habitat

Rosemary grows as a bush on dry scrub land on the hillsides of southern Mediterranean countries.

Season

Rosemary is an evergreen plant, but it puts out fresh green shoots in the spring and tiny flowers in the summer.

Cultivation

Rosemary needs a sunny position and light well drained soil. It thrives during long, hot summers and can withstand periods of drought. The stems thicken with time and can eventually form a substantial trunk but the new growth is soft and flexible. To propagate, cut pieces of new growth, around 10 cm long, in early to midsummer and insert them into a pot of compost. Keep them moist and they should root by the autumn, when you can pot them up and grow them on before planting out in spring.

Parts Used

The leaves.

Preservation

It is better to use rosemary fresh if you possibly can.

Properties

Rosemary is diuretic, antiseptic, astringent and wound healing. It is antidepressant, tonic and calms the nerves. It is aromatic, helps to relieve gas, stimulates the liver and digestion and relaxes the smooth muscle of the intestines. Extract of rosemary relaxes the smooth muscles of the trachea and makes a dry cough productive. Rosemary is rich in volatile oils, flavonoids and phenolic acids, which are antiseptic, antifungal and anti-inflammatory. It contains caffeic acid and its derivatives, such as rosmarinic acid, which are antioxidant. Rosmarinic acid relaxes the muscles of the trachea, the bronchi and the intestine and inhibits some of the enzymes linked with memory loss. According to Duke rosmarol, another compound from rosemary, is highly antioxidant. The German Commission E Monographs approve *Rosmarinus officinalis* rosemary for rheumatism, indigestion, loss of appetite and blood pressure problems.

Chemical Constituents

There are at least 33 compounds in the essential oil of rosemary, including esters, largely as borneol; cineoles and several terpenes, chiefly pinene and camphene, camphor, verbenone, borneol, piperitone, limonene and thymol. Hoefler and Wu also identified rosmarol, rosmarinic acid and chlorogenic acid. Oluwatuyi in 2004 identified several diterpenes, including carnosolic acid and carnosol which are antibacterial. Houlihan identified rosmaridiphenol, rosmariquinone and many other natural antioxidants. Kotb identified ursolic acid, glucocolic acid and the alkaloid rosmaricine.

Research

There has been a great deal of research into the healing properties of rosemary, much of which was carried out in the laboratory. In 1987 Kimura demonstrated that rosmarinic acid increased the production of prostaglandin E2, which stimulates the bronchi to dilate, while it reduced leukotrienes, which cause the bronchi to constrict, so it may help people suffering from asthma. Since leukotrienes are also involved in rheumatism and rheumatoid arthritis, rosemary may well help these conditions too. In 1999 al Sereiti and his team in India demonstrated that rosmarinic acid is responsible for this effect.

Herbs such as rosemary, sage, onion, thyme and garlic, much used in Mediterranean cooking, contain large quantities of water-soluble phenolic acids and flavonoids, that can scavenge reactive oxygen and protect us from inflammation and cancer. Many different scientists, including Singletary in 1991, have investigated the anticancer effects of rosemary. Singletary demonstrated that rosemary extract prevented breast cancer in rats. In 2011 Suong reviewed the scientific evidence that rosemary protects people from various kinds of cancer. He found that rosemary extract and the rosemary compounds: carnosol, carnosic acid, ursolic acid and rosmarinic acid, all have anti-cancer effects. Rosemary compounds prevent tumours from developing in several organs, including colon, breast, liver and stomach, as well as in melanoma and leukaemia cells. In 2011 Johnson reviewed the research on the anti-cancer properties of carnosol, a diterpene flavonoid from rosemary. It selectively kills prostate, breast, skin, leukemia and colon cancer cells. Several scientists have investigated the anti-cancer effects of carnosol, including Huang in 1994, who demonstrated that both rosemary extract and carnosol inhibited a cell division promoter and prevented tumours from developing in mouse skin. Carnosol is also anti-oxidant and anti-inflammatory, according to Lo in 2002. Oxidative stress and inflammation can both cause cancer, so anti-oxidant, anti-inflammatory compounds help to prevent cancer.

Oxidation of low density lipoproteins (bad fats) contributes to the development of atherosclerosis, hardening of the arteries and several degenerative disorders that afflict old people, according to Schwarz in 2001. In 1984 Rulffs demonstrated that rosemary oil in the bath stimulates the skin, improves circulation and improves blood flow in people suffering from hardening of the arteries. Mediterranean diets which include considerable amounts of garlic, rosemary, basil and thyme, among other herbs, provide sufficient flavonoids to prevent the oxidation of LDL and thus protect the walls of the arteries. This may help to explain why people living in Mediterranean countries have fewer degenerative disorders, including heart disease, and live such long and healthy lives.

The gram-negative bacterium *Helicobacter pylori* is one of the main causes of gastritis, peptic ulcer, gastric carcinoma and gastric B-cell lymphoma. In 2005 Mahady demonstrated that rosemary extract killed *Helicobacter*. In 1991 Aqel demonstrated that rosemary volatile oil stopped the smooth muscle of the trachea of rabbits and guinea pigs from contracting. In 1992 Al-Sereiti found that rosemary leaf extract inhibited rabbit jejunum contractions. If rosemary has a similar calming effect on the human gut, it could help to cure gastritis and peptic ulcer. In 1987 Hoefler found that the rosemary extracts protected rats' livers.

Many different scientists have demonstrated that rosemary extracts and essential oil are antibacterial. Pintore, in 2002, identified fifty-eight compounds in *Rosmarinus officinalis* L. essential oil from Sardinia and Corsica. He found that it took sixty minutes for the essential oil to completely kill several different bacteria. In 2007 Yesil Celiktas and his team collected rosemary from three different regions of Turkey, at four different times of the year, made extracts and distilled essential oil from these samples. They found that the essential oils destroyed several different bacteria and fungi and were more or less potent according to which location they came from and what time of the year they were harvested. In 2005 Santoyo identified 33 compounds in rosemary essential oil, including α-pinene, 1,8-cineole, camphor, verbenone, and borneol. He also demonstrated that it killed bacteria, yeast and fungi. In 2007 Bozin demonstrated that rosemary essential oil inhibited thirteen different bacteria and six fungi, including *Candida albicans* and the essential oil was antioxidant. In 2004 Oluwatuyi demonstrated that several rosemary diterpenes helped erythromycin to kill multi-drug resistant bacteria. These bacteria usually survive by pumping antibiotics out of their cells and the rosemary diterpenes interfered with this pumping mechanism.

The fungus, *Aspergillus,* which sometimes infects food, produces Aflatoxin B1, which is highly toxic and carcinogenic. In 2008 Rasooli found that rosemary essential oil stopped *Aspergillus parasiticus* from producing Aflatoxin. He identified piperitone, α-pinene, limonene, 1, 8-cineole and thymol in the essential oil, each or all of which may have been responsible for the anti-fungal effect.

Rosemary has long had a reputation for stimulating memory and in 1987 Kovar demonstrated that rosemary oil stimulated mice to become active and stimulated their brains. In 2009 Machado found that rosemary extract had an anti-depressant effect in mice. In 2003 Kosaka demonstrated *in vitro* that the rosemary compound, carnosic acid, stimulates the synthesis of nerve growth factor, which is vital for the growth and maintenance of nerves. In 2008 Orhan tested rosemary extracts and essential oil from Turkey on the enzymes acetylcholinesterase and butyryl-cholinesterase. He found that the extracts, the essential oil and rosemarinic acid inhibited these enzymes. Acetylcholinesterase and butyrylcholinesterase break down acetylcholine, a chemical messenger which sends signals to the muscles and the brain. Acetylcholine plays an important role in the arousal, attention, memory and motivation areas of the brain. The medical profession uses acetylcholinesterase inhibitors to treat Alzheimer's disease. But these have severe side effects, do not stop the disease from progressing and may not be appropriate until the patient has reached an advanced stage of the disease. Rosemary appears to stop acetylcholine from being broken down, which results in these areas of the brain being stimulated for longer without the damaging side effects of conventional medication. In 2012 Pengelly carried out a randomised, placebo controlled double blind clinical trial to investigate the effects of rosemary leaf powder on the cognitive function of twenty-eight people with a mean age of 75. Lower doses of rosemary (750 mg) speeded up the patients' memory but higher doses (6000 mg) made their memory worse. 750 mg is approximately the amount that people add to food in Mediterranean countries.

In 1997 Matsunaga showed that an extract of *R officinalis* had an antidepressant effect on mice. In 1998 Diego carried out a study on forty human adults to assess brain activity, alertness and mood after three minutes of aromatherapy, with lavender or rosemary. The lavender group showed increased beta power, were less depressed and felt more relaxed performing maths computations faster and accurately. The rosemary group was more alert, less anxious and faster but not accurate at the maths computations. In 2005 Atsumi carried out a clinical trial on 22 healthy volunteers, who sniffed rosemary and lavender aroma for five minutes. He collected their saliva and measured the free radical scavenging activity in it. Both lavender and rosemary stimulation caused the stress hormone, cortisol to decrease.

In 1979 Durakovic treated cancer patients suffering from *Candida* which nystatin had failed to cure. He put a cotton swab soaked in an emulsion of rosemary oil and water (1:10) in the patients' mouths, five times a day. The *Candida* disappeared completely in 2-4 days.

In 1998 Hay tested a combination of essential oils, including rosemary oil, in a randomized, double-blind, controlled trial of

84 patients suffering from alopecia areata, spot baldness. Alopecia areata is an autoimmune disease in which the patient loses patches of hair due to the body's failure to recognise its own body cells, so that it destroys them. He gave the active test group a combination of essential oils from thyme, *Thymus vulgaris* (88 mg), lavender, *Lavandula angustifoli*a (108 mg), rosemary (*Rosmarinus officinalis* 114 mg), and cedar, *Cedrus atlantica* (94 mg), mixed in a carrier oil of 3 ml jojoba oil and 20 ml grape seed oil. The control group used the carrier oils. Both groups massaged the oils into their scalps for two minutes each night and wrapped a warm towel around their heads. The treatment group improved significantly, there were no side effects and the treatment was just as effective as other available treatments for alopecia.

In Jordan people traditionally use rosemary to treat wounds. So in 2010 Abu-Al-Basal demonstrated that the essential oil of rosemary helped diabetic wounds to heal in mice. In 2000 Calabrese found that rosemary extract was strongly antioxidant on men's skin. It prevented skin surface lipids from being oxidised so he suggested that it could be used in anti-ageing treatments for the skin.

Some opium addicts do not want to continue treatment because they cannot bear the withdrawal symptoms, so in 2013 Solhi and his team evaluated rosemary, in addition to therapy, to alleviate withdrawal symptoms. They divided eighty-one patients into case and control groups. They treated the case group with methadone and powdered dried leaves of *Rosmarinus officinalis* for four weeks. They treated the control group with methadone and placebo for the same interval. They found that patients in the case group experienced less severe withdrawal syndrome (bone pain, perspiration and insomnia) compared to those in the control group. They suggested that rosemary could be used as an optional extra to treat withdrawal symptoms during treatment programs for opium addiction.

How to Use

Above all, use rosemary in food as often as you can. The great thing about rosemary is that you can pick it from a bush growing in your garden (if you have one) at any time of the year. But if you don't have a garden supermarkets now sell fresh rosemary, which you can add to fish, meat or beans, or chop it up finely and add it to stuffings and sauces. Add rosemary to olive oil and leave to macerate for weeks. This will add a delightful flavour to your salad dressing. Roast vegetables are infinitely improved by the addition of rosemary. Add rosemary to soups. If you bake bread try adding sun-dried tomatoes, finely chopped rosemary and chopped onions to your dough for a Mediterranean flavoured bread.

Use an infusion for colds, coughs, influenza, indigestion, rheumatic pain, headaches, colic, depression and as an antispasmodic in renal colic and menstrual pain. Use it to relieve flatulence, stomach cramps, constipation and bloating. Use it to stimulate the liver and gall bladder. It will help to regulate the release of bile which will aid digestion and improve the absorption of nutrients from food. Use as a mouth wash to sweeten your breath, remove bacteria and prevent gingivitis.

Dilute the essential oil in a carrier oil to massage aching joints. Use on the skin as an antiseptic and to heal wounds, to cure eczema, dermatitis, oily skin and acne. Add rosemary essential oil to face creams and moisturisers to tone your skin. Rosemary oil and rosemary infusion help to stimulate hair follicles, if you use them regularly, making hair grow longer and stronger and slowing down premature hair loss. Rosemary massage oil, made with olive oil, nourishes the scalp and removes dandruff. Use rosemary essential oil vapour to lift your spirits, stimulate your brain, calm your nerves and improve concentration. It is a good remedy for depression, mental fatigue and forgetfulness.

Use relaxing, calming rosemary aromatherapy to de-stress.

Dose

Make an infusion of 5-10 grams of the flowering stems of rosemary per litre of boiled water in a closed container to prevent the steam from escaping.

Fluid extracts (1:1, 45 % ethanol v/v): 1.5-3 ml daily.

Tincture (1:5, 70 % ethanol): 3-8.5 ml daily.

Use the essential oils of rosemary: 3 to 4 drops, 3-4 times/day mixed with a carrier oil.

Contraindications

Fresh rosemary leaves in food and as an infusion are quite safe. The essential oil of rosemary is potent and should not be taken internally in large doses since it may cause gastrointestinal and kidney disturbances. Essential oil of rosemary can irritate the skin, if it hasn't been adequately diluted with a carrier oil. You should not take phenolic-rich extracts of rosemary long term because they reduce the uptake of dietary iron. Pregnant and breastfeeding women should not use it.

Chapter 7

Sage *Salvia officinalis*

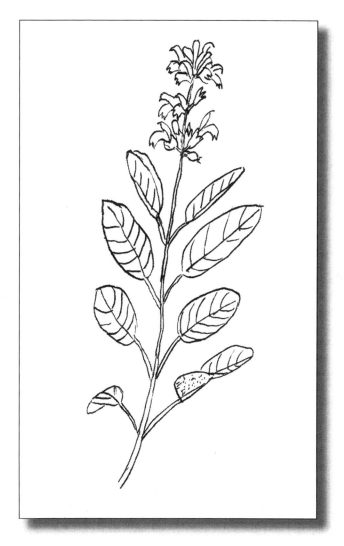

I have a huge sage plant growing in my garden. Every year it threatens to take over the path and I hack it back brutally, sometimes putting the cut branches on top of my wood burning stove to release the wonderful smell as the leaves heat up and begin to shrivel. I give away masses of it and throw the rest of the leaves in the compost, carefully stripped off the woody part. The slow worms, slugs, toads and all the other creatures in my compost seem to love it. I don't need to store sage because I can simply pick some leaves off the bush whenever I need them.

The Romans discovered sage in Egypt, adopted it and later brought it to Britain when they invaded. The ancient Celts adopted it and we in Britain have been growing sage in our gardens ever since. Over the centuries the cultivation of sage has spread throughout the world, including the US.

Salvia comes from the Latin *salvere*, to save; and the ancient Greeks, Egyptians and Romans used it medicinally. *Salvia* is one of the widest-spread members of the Labiatae family; it features prominently in the pharmacopoeas of many countries from the Far East, through Europe and across the Americas. There are almost one thousand different *Salvia* species, which people have been using traditionally for centuries to treat a multitude of different symptoms. Most of these species have medicinal properties, but I am going to focus on *Salvia officinalis*.

According to Mrs Grieve there is an old tradition that Rue should be planted among the sage, to keep away noxious toads from the valued, cherished plants. People believed that the sage plant would thrive or wither, just as the owner's business prospered or failed, and in Buckinghamshire another tradition maintained that the wife rules when sage grows vigorously in the garden. People believed that sage would ward off evil and dispel evil spirits.

In the Jura district of France, people believe that sage mitigates grief, mental and bodily, and Pepys in his diary says: 'Between Gosport and Southampton we observed a little churchyard where it was customary to sow all the graves with sage.' Gerard said: 'No man need to doubt of the wholesomeness of sage ale, being brewed as it should be with sage, betony, scabious, spikenard, squinnette (squinancywort) and fennell seed.'

In ancient Egypt they used it as a fertility drug and Dioscorides advised people to make a decoction of sage leaves to stop wounds bleeding and to clean ulcers and sores. Sage has a long history of use as a treatment for sore throats, coughs and colds.

Turkey is one of the most important sage producing countries in the world. They produce approximately 500 kg of sage leaf oil from *Salvia triloba* every year and export 600 tonnes of sage leaves. People in Turkey used to collect so much wild sage that they threatened to make the native sage extinct; so now it is grown commercially.

Botanical Description

Salvia officinalis is a perennial plant that grows up to three feet high as a dense bush, with blue/violet flowers in the summer. The leaves grow in pairs on the stem and are one to one and a half inches long, with stalks, oblong, rounded at the ends, finely wrinkled by a strongly-marked network of greyish-green veins on both sides, softly hairy and glandular underneath. The flowers are in whorls and the corollas lipped. The whole plant has a strong scent and a warm, bitter, astringent taste, due to the volatile oil in it.

Habitat

Sage is native to the southern Mediterranean, from Spain along the Mediterranean coast up to and including the east side of the Adriatic; it grows mostly where there is a limestone formation with very little soil. Wild sage has a more penetrating smell than the plants we grow in our gardens.

Season

Sage flowers in August.

How to Grow

You can grow sage from seed but it is easier to take cuttings of the young shoots of a three-year-old plant in spring, towards the end of April, as soon as they are hard enough to stick into the ground, or into potting compost. Sage likes a well drained soil, grows well in stony ground and tolerates drought well. It likes a nice sunny position.

Parts Used

The leaves.

Preservation

Sage is best used fresh, when you will benefit from all the essential oils in the leaves but you can also dry the leaves to use when you are not near to a growing plant. Pick the leaves before the plant begins to flower and dry them in a warm, airy place away from the sun.

Properties

Sage is stimulant, astringent, tonic and carminative, so it is good for dyspepsia. Sage tea has a calming effect on sweat glands and reduces outbreaks of sweat. Since it is mildly oestrogenic and mood enhancing the tea helps to allay the symptoms of menopause and pre-menstrual syndrome. It contains phenolic acids which are antibacterial and makes an excellent cough mixture, when mixed with lemon juice and honey. Sage infusion used as a gargle will sooth tonsillitis, laryngitis and bronchitis and help them to heal. Sage is also antioxidant and anti-inflammatory.

Chemical Constituents

Scientists all over the world have investigated the chemical constituents of sage. Lu and Yeap Foo in 2002 reviewed the chemistry of the polyphenols in all the different species of sage. From their review you can see that many species of sage contain compounds that have healing properties. I am focussing on *Salvia officinalis,* the species that the Romans brought to Britain, which is a rich source of polyphenols; more than one hundred and sixty have been identified. Caffeic acid is the central building block of the polyphenols in sage. Two caffeic acids together form rosmarinic acid which is highly antioxidant. Three and four caffeic acids form trimers and tetramers such as salvianolic acids and lithospermic acid, which are powerful free radical scavengers. Sage contains phenolic acids such as ursolic acid, which is anti-inflammatory. It contains phenolic glucosides and glycosides of neolignans. It contains flavonoids, such as the oestrogenic luteolin-7-O-glucoside. Most of the flavonoids are flavones of apigenin and luteolin or flavonols such as kaempferol and quercetin; methyl ethers and their glycosides. It also contains methyl ethers of flavones in the leaves or in the exudate from aerial parts. It contains quercetin glycosides and their methyl ethers. *Salvia officinalis* contains proanthocyanidins, or condensed tannins. It also contains essential oil, composed of at least sixty-eight different compounds, which is anti-bacterial, according to Hayouni in 2008. The main components are thujone, viriflorol, manool, caryophylene and humulene. It contains the cyclic monoterpenes, 1, 8-cineol, pinene and camphor, which inhibit acetylcholinesterase.

Research

There has been masses of research into the healing properties of sage and, yet again, it would not be appropriate for me to attempt to cover it all.

Several different scientists, including Longaray Delamare in 2007, have demonstrated that sage essential oil inhibited and/or killed a number of different bacteria. In 2007 Pinto found that essential oil which he had distilled from *Salvia officinalis* inhibited fungi and yeasts, including *Candida.*

In 2001 Saller carried out a clinical study on patients with lip sores caused by *Herpes simplex*. He gave the patients a cream containing sage and rhubarb to rub onto the sores. It helped relieve the pain and swelling. The sores went more quickly when the sage/rhubarb cream was rubbed on than without treatment.

A great many scientists have investigated the antioxidant, anti-inflammatory and sedative effects of sage. In 2001 Baricevic found that the anti-inflammatory effect of *Salvia officinalis* leaves was due to ursolic acid, which is twice as potent as indomethacin. In 2007 Reuter carried out a randomised, double-blind, placebo-controlled study to investigate the anti-inflammatory effects of a sage extract on erythema (redness) caused by ultraviolet light. He irradiated test areas on the backs of healthy volunteers then treated them with 2% sage ointment. He treated the controls with hydrocortisone ointment or with a placebo ointment. The sage ointment reduced the inflammation as much as the hydrocortisone ointment did, which was significantly more than the placebo.

High levels of fats in the bloodstream contribute to heart disease, atherosclerosis and deterioration of the brain. Conventional drugs to reduce fats in the bloodstream sometimes have severe side effects and only work to a limited extent. Sage leaves inhibit the oxidation and absorption of fats, so numerous scientists, including Kianbakht in 2011, have demonstrated that sage reduces fats in the bloodstream. Kianbakht carried out a double blind, placebo controlled clinical trial with sixty-seven patients who all had high fats, high cholesterol or high triglycerides in their bloodstream. He gave them a 500 mg capsule of sage leaf extract every eight hours for 2 months. He found that the extract lowered blood levels of the fats, cholesterol and triglycerides in the patients who took the sage leaf compared with the placebo. Then in 2013 he carried out another clinical trial with sage, this time with type two diabetic patients who had high cholesterol and/or high triglycerides in their bloodstreams. This time he measured glucose levels in their blood as well as cholesterol and triglycerides. He found that the extract lowered glucose, choles-terol and triglycerides in the blood of the patients who took the sage, compared with those who took the placebo. Several other scientists, including Behradmanesh in 2013 have demonstrated that sage lowers blood sugar and cholesterol in diabetic patients.

There has been a great deal of interest in the beneficial effect of sage on Alzheimer's disease. In 2003 Akhondzadeh carried out a four-month clinical trial on forty-two patients in Iran with mild to moderate Alzheimer's. He gave the patients either *Salvia officinalis* extract or a placebo. The patients who took the sage extract were less agitated and their memory and understanding was significantly better than that of the patients who took the placebo. In 2008 Scholey carried out a similar randomised, pla-cebo-controlled, double-blind study on 65-90-year-old healthy adults. He also found that the people who took a 333 mg dose of sage extract had improved secondary memory.

Scientists think that Alzheimer's disease is due in part to in-flammation and damage to the brain cells caused by compounds which oxidise fats. Acetylcholine is a neurotransmitter involved in brain activity. It plays an important role in the arousal, at-tention, memory and motivation areas of the brain and acetyl-cholinesterase is the enzyme that breaks it down. Alzheimer pa-tients are often given acetylcholinesterase inhibitors, which have serious side effects and do not alter the long term progress of the disease. Several scientists, including Haughton in 2004, found that various monoterpenoids from sage, including the cyclic monoterpenes: 1, 8-cineol, alpha-pinene and camphor inhibit cholinesterase. This allows acetylcholine to continue to stimu-late those parts of the brain which are affected by Alzheimer's and thus improve memory and understanding.

In 2006 Kennedy carried out a double-blind, placebo-con-trolled, crossover study on thirty healthy young people (average age 24 years). First he made an extract of dried sage leaf, then demonstrated that it inhibited acetylcholinesterase, which has the effect of reducing negative mood and anxiety. Kennedy gave the participants 600 or 300 mg of dried sage leaf or placebo, then he assessed their mood. He also made the participants perform on a Defined Intensity Stress Simulator (DISS). Their mood improved with both doses when they didn't use the stressor. When they took 300 mg they became less anxious and when they took 600 mg they became more alert, calm and contented. When they performed on the stressor while taking 600 mg of sage leaf they were less anxious and more alert. But when they performed on it while taking 300 mg they were more anxious and less alert.

In 2010 Moss gave five drops of essential oils of *Salvia officinalis* or *Salvia lavandulifolia* or placebo in 5 ml of water to 135 healthy adults. The *Salvia officinalis* group performed significantly better than the *Salvia lavandulifolia* and control groups. Their long-term or secondary memory was better while their working was not affected.

There has been a lot of interest in the oestrogenic effects of sage. Dysmenorrhea (painful menstruation) includes symptoms such as menstrual cramps, headache, fatigue, nausea, vomiting and diarrhoea. Doctors sometimes treat dysmenorrhea with pain relievers, sedatives, antispasmodics, prostaglandin inhibitors and oral contraceptives. All these drugs produce unacceptable side effects. In 2006 Han carried out a survey of sixty-seven female college students in Korea and found that 83% experience menstrual cramps and nearly 20% describe their menstrual pain as severe. Various essential oils help menstrual symptoms and are absorbed through the skin, so Han gave fifteen minutes of abdominal massage with the essential oils of lavender (2 drops), clary sage (*Salvia sclarea*) (one drop) and rose (*Rosa centifolia*) (one drop), mixed in almond oil every day for a week before menstruation, ending on the first day of menstruation. He gave the placebo group abdominal massage with almond oil, and no massage at all to the control group. The intensity of the menstrual cramps on both the first and second days of menstruation was significantly lower in the group receiving the essential oil massage than in the placebo group or the control group. I wonder whether *Salvia officinalis* essential oil would have the same effect as *Salvia sclarea*.

In 1998 De Leo carried out a clinical trial giving extracts of *Salvia officinalis* and alfalfa (*Medicago sativa*) to thirty menopausal women suffering from hot flushes, insomnia, nocturnal sweating, dizziness, headaches and palpitations. Twenty of these women reported that their hot flushes and night sweating had completely disappeared. Four women said that their symptoms improved a lot and the remaining six said that their symptoms improved a little. In 2013 Rahte isolated and identified luteolin-7-O-glucoside from *Salvia officinalis,* an oestrogenic flavonoid which he believed was responsible for the reduction in frequency and intensity of the menopausal hot flushes, but the De Leo trial also included alfalfa, which has oestrogenic properties.

How to Use

There are many ways to use sage. You can chew whole fresh sage leaves to strengthen your gums, or dry the leaves and grind them with sea salt into a powder to clean your teeth. You can steep them in boiling water to make an infusion or boil them to make a decoction. Herbalists use sage tincture, which preserves most of the properties of the herb. Make an ointment by heating sage leaves in oil, then straining it and adding wax. Use the ointment on cold sores. Put sage leaves in your bath to treat varicose veins, leg ulcers, wounds, sores and eczema.

Use an infusion of fresh or dried leaves for indigestion, inflammation of the mouth and throat. Take sage infusion or tea to calm premenstrual tension, menopausal symptoms such as irritation, sleeplessness and night sweats. Drink the infusion to cleanse and purify the blood. Massage the infusion of sage and rosemary into your scalp to encourage your hair to grow. The German Commission E approved the use of sage tea or decoction for indigestion, heartburn, bloating, excessive perspiration and for inflammation of the nose and throat. Use for gum inflammations, sore mouth and throat and for pressure spots caused by prostheses. Give frequent doses of sage tea to patients suffering from delirium when they have a fever. Give sage tea to patients suffering from nervous conditions, trembling, depression and vertigo. It helps to calm the nervous excitement that often accompanies brain and nervous diseases such as Alzheimer's. Rub sage ointment onto the skin to ease muscular pain, for sciatica and for loosening stiff and painful joints. Wilt the leaves in hot water and use as a poultice on stings and bites.

Of course sage is a wonderful culinary herb that you can use in stuffings, sauces, with potatoes, meats, in nut roasts, in omelettes, with white beans, as sage butter on gnocchi or ravioli, sage butter on trout, with olive oil on pasta, in risottos, prosciutto and sage involtini, butternut squash with sage and so on. There are hundreds of Italian recipes that use sage, one of the most delicious being sage and lemon sorbet. Eat sage every day to improve your memory and concentration and prevent the mental deterioration that so often accompanies old age.

Plant sage in your vegetable garden to keep insect pests away.

I would not recommend using sage essential oil as it is too strong and even the smell of it can cause intoxication and giddiness.

Dose

4-6 g of leaf.
2.5-7.5 g/day of alcoholic extract.
1.8-3.0 g/day of fluid extract.
Infusion: 30g of dried sage to one pint of boiling water. Drink half a teacupful as often as required.

Contraindications

Do not take the essential oil of sage. It can cause convulsions. It is too strong to use even in aromatherapy, unless greatly diluted. Avoid sage during pregnancy since it stimulates the uterus to contract. Do not use sage while breastfeeding, since it will cause your milk to dry up.

Lessons to Be Learned from the Ancient Celts

The ancient Celts lived in harmony with their environment, in much the same way as native, tribal people the world over still do today. They revered every aspect of it, the trees, the rivers and springs, the rock formations, the animals and birds who shared their world and this reverence engendered respect and awe. They knew that their environment provided them with everything they needed, food, water, shelter and medicine. Most of Britain was covered with thick forest, which they did not attempt to tame. They built their settlements on the tops of hills and cleared small areas around them, just big enough to till the land needed to grow food. They lived in close contact with nature, teaching their children to recognise plants that were edible, plants to use as medicine and plants that were poisonous.

The Druids of the ancient Celts were shamanic priests who performed ceremonies, healed the sick and formed a network of wise men and women, guardians of the spirits of the land, lawmakers and advisors to the kings and queens of the various tribes. Right up until the Roman invasion women had the same rights as men, were taken seriously and listened to. It is time that we women remember that we are wise women and use the wonderful healing plants that the earth provides us with to keep ourselves, our families and friends healthy. It is time to treat all those little ailments, like coughs, colds and sore throats, safely and effectively, rather than taking pharmaceutical drugs. It is time that we take back control of our health and well-being.

Most of us in the West have lost touch with our environment, living in urban conglomerations, surrounded by buildings, tarmac and fast-moving vehicles. Our children no longer recognise the native plants that grow in the countryside or the many different species of trees that provide us with oxygen, soak up the rain and retain the soil, although many of these trees grow in our city parks.

But many of us in Britain have small gardens, where we can grow some of the herbs we need to heal ourselves. There are often allotments in the big cities, available for a small fee, where we can grow vegetables, fruit and herbs. We should learn from the ancient Celts to spend as much time in the natural environment as possible, learning the names of as many plants as we can, teaching our children to recognise the plants that provide us with food and medicine, the names of the different species of trees. If children cannot be brought up in the country they can visit the parks, collect the falling leaves in the autumn, learn about the trees that the leaves come from, draw pictures of them, make leaf patterns and play with them in all sorts of different ways. Ideally schools, especially inner city schools, should have vegetable gardens, where children can learn how to grow vegetables and herbs from seed.

Another important lesson we can learn from the ancient Celts is that overeating leads to ill health. The Physicians of Myddfai recommend:

> Whosoever would prolong life, should restrain his appetite, and not eat over abundantly.
>
> Whosoever, restraining their appetite, refrain from gluttony and eat slowly, these shall live long.

It is important to eat slowly, pausing between mouthfuls, chewing each mouthful well. People who eat fast tend to eat more than people who eat slowly. Mealtimes should be important social occasions, where people meet together to converse and enjoy their food. People who eat in front of a TV or some other screen, such as the office computer, are unaware of what they are eating, how much they eat or how fast they eat it.

'If you eat simple food it will be more easy for the stomach to digest it.'

Of course processed food did not exist at the time of the ancient Celts, but processed food exemplifies the kind of food that you should not eat. Simple food means fruit, vegetables, grains, pulses, nuts, eggs, all grown organically and simply cooked or eaten raw in salads, with maybe a little fish or meat occasionally.

The ancient Celts did not have sugar and honey was a luxury, eaten on rare occasions or used to make mead. Recent research suggests that sugar is as bad for you as saturated fat. Of course we all know that sugar is bad for our teeth but we tend to forget that it is harmful to the rest of our bodies as well. It is absorbed into the blood so fast that it stimulates the pancreas to secrete insulin, which takes the sugar out of the blood and stores it as fat. This leaves the bloodstream without sugar, so that you immediately crave more sugar. These swings between high and low blood sugar cause mood swings, fatigue and increase the risk of obesity, diabetes and heart disease, according to Bell in 2003. Excess sugar may even contribute to loss of elasticity of the skin and signs of ageing, according to Sensi in 1991, as well as causing bacteria and yeast to breed and multiply, resulting in conditions such as Candidiasis. As if all this were not enough, according to USDA data people who eat the most sugar consume the least vitamins (A, C, B12, folate) and minerals (calcium, phosphorous, magnesium and iron).

'When you eat, do not eat away all your appetite but let some desire for food remain.'

'Do not eat, till the stomach has become empty.'

This is very important. Many people eat out of habit, rather than waiting until they feel hungry.

People who overeat risk having high levels of fats in their blood stream, becoming obese and developing type two diabetes, high blood pressure, hardening of the arteries and heart disease. Cardiovascular disease is the leading cause of ill health and death in the US and is rapidly increasing in Britain. But it can be prevented and even reversed by eating less, more healthily and by taking regular exercise. The Baltimore Longitudinal Study of Aging found that people who eat less live longer, have healthier hearts and fewer disabling diseases than people who gain weight. The people who lived the longest in the study were the ones who lost weight as they aged and decreased the calories they consumed as they gradually became less active. At the time of the USDA study the rest of the population in the US were eating more and more carbohydrate and fat. Restricting the amount of calories you eat but making sure you eat a balanced diet seems to slow down the ageing process of the heart and blood vessels and prevent cardiac and arterial stiffness and heart rate variability, possibly by preventing inflammation and oxidative stress. Eating less protects the heart from fibrosis, protects against obesity, diabetes, high blood pressure and cancer. It keeps you healthier for longer and improves the quality of your life.

The Physicians of Myddvai advised people to drink plenty of spring water for its miraculous health-giving qualities. There was no tea or coffee at the time of the ancient Celts and although they brewed mead and a few were able to import wine, they did not drink alcohol on a regular basis but only during the many festivals throughout the year. Water protectors have drawn attention to the importance of pure water, giver of life to humans, animals and plants. In Italy people travel miles with their containers to collect water from springs whose qualities they particularly enjoy. Ideally we should only drink water, though an occasional cup of tea or coffee or glass of wine does no harm. We should certainly never drink sugary carbonated drinks, which add empty calories and rot our teeth.

So although we cannot return to living in the natural environment of the ancient Celts, we can certainly benefit from their sage advice to eat simple food, only when we are hungry, to drink plenty of pure water, to exercise regularly and above all to be aware of our natural environment, live in harmony with it, respect every aspect of it and use the healing plants it provides.

References

Introduction

Aldhouse-Green M. 2000. Seeing the Wood for the Trees: Symbolism of Trees and Wood in Ancient Gaul and Britain. Aberystwyth: Centres for Advanced Welsh and Celtic Studies. University of Wales, Aberystwyth Research Paper No 17.

Aldhouse-Green M. 2006. Boudica Britannia; Routledge.

Andouze and Buchsenschutz 1991. Towns, Villages and Countryside of Celtic Europe, Translated Henry Cleere BCA.

Caesar J. translated by WA Mc Devitte and WS Bohn 1869. Commentaries on the Gallic War. Harper and Brothers New York.

Champlin E. 1991. Final Judgements: Deity and Emotion in Roman Wills, 200 BC-AD 250. Berkley: University of California Press.

Cunliffe B 2002. The Extraordinary Voyage of Pytheas the Greek. Penguin.

Del Pozo 1979. Empiricism and Magic in Aztec Pharmacology. From Ethno-Pharmacologic Search for Psychoactive Drugs, Raven Press.

Fox 1958. Pattern and Purpose: A survey of Celtic Art in Britain. Cardiff.

Graves R. 1948. The White Goddess: a Historical Grammar of Poetic Myth. Faber and Faber.

Grimes WF 1961. Some Smaller Settlements: A Symposium. Problems of the Iron Age in Southern Britain: 25-8.

Hutton R. 2007. The Druids. Hambledon Continuum.

Hutton R. 2009. Blood and Mistletoe. The History of the Druids in Britain. Yale University Press.

Jacobsthal P 1944. Early Celtic Art. Oxford. Two vols.

Kennedy M. Silchester Iron Age Finds Reveal Secrets of pre-Roman Britain. Guardian 31 July 2012

Koch. J.T. 2013 Tartessian: Celtic in the South-west at the Dawn of History, Celtic Studies Publications 13, Aberystwyth, pp. xii + 332. Revised & expanded edition. 978–1–891271–19–9 First edition published 2009.

Koch. J.T. 2014. Co-editor and contributing author, Celtic from the West. Alternative Perspectives from Archaeology, Genetics, Language, and Literature. Oxford: Oxbow Books, pp. viii + 388.

Lucan. Pharsalia I. 4: 50-8

Markale J 1975. Women of the Celts, Translated by A Mygind, C Hauch and P Henry. Gordon Cremonesi.

Matthews C and J 1994. Encyclopaedia of Celtic Wisdom. A Celtic Shaman's Source Book. Element.

Miles D 2005. The Tribes of Britain. Phoenix,

Pelletier A 1984. La Femme dans la Société Gallo-Romaine. Paris, Picard.

Pezron, P. 1703. Antiquite de la Nation, et de la Langue des Celtes, autrement appellez les Gaulois. Pub: Jean Boudot; Paris.

Pliny Historiae Naturalis.

Ross A. 1967. Pagan Celtic Britain. Studies in Iconography and Tradition. Rutledge and Kegan Paul.

Sjoestedt ML 1926. Le Siege de Druim Damhghaire. Rev. Celt. XL III: 1-12.

Stokes 1894. The Prose tales in the Rennes Dindshenchas. Rev Celt XV 272-336. 418-84

Strabo, 23 AD Geographica.

The Physicians of Myddvai Translated by John Pughe. 1993 Llanerch.

Williamson WC 1872. Description of the Tumuli opened at Gristhorpe near Scarborough.

Zethelius M and Balick MJ 1982. Modern medicine and shamanistic ritual: a case of positive synergistic response in the treatment of a snakebite. J Ethnopharmacol 5.181-185.

Part II

Chapter 1 Betony

Ahmad, VU et al. 2006. New phenethyl alcohol glycosides from *Stachys parviflora*. J Asian Nat Prod. Res. 8 (1-2) 105-111.

Haznagy-Radnai et al. 2012. Anti-inflammatory activities of Hungarian *Stachys* species and their iridoids. Phytotherapy Research 26 (4) 505-509.

Marin PD et al 2004. Glycosides of tricetin methyl ethers as chemo-systematic markers in *Stachys* subgenus *Betonica*. Phytochemistry 65; 1247-1253.

Matkowski A and Piotrowska M 2006. Antioxidant and free radical scavenging activities of some medicinal plants from the Lamiaceae. Fitoterpia 77 (5) 346-53

Peleshchuk AP et al. 1974. Stachyglen treatment of patients with chronic cholecystitis and cholangitis. Vrachebnoe delo 1:65-69.

Rabbani M et al. 2003. Anxiolytic effects of *Stachys lavandulifolia* Vahl on the elevated plus-maze model of anxiety in mice. J Ethnopharmacol 2003; 89 (2-3): 271-276.

Schofield C. www.naturesbestmedicine.info

Skaltsa et al. 2000. Inhibition of prostaglandin E2 and leukotriene C4 in mouse peritoneal macrophages and thromboxane B2 production in human platelets by flavonoids from *Stachys chrysantha* and *Stachys candida*. Biol Pharm Bull 2000; 23 (1); 47-53

Skaltsa et al. 2003. Essential oil analysis and antimicrobial activity of eight *Stachys* species from Greece Phytochemistry 64:743-752.

Stamatis G et al. 2003. *In vitro* anti-*Helicobacter pylori* activity of Greek herbal medicines. Journal of Ethnopharmacology 88:175-179.

Vundac et al. 2007. Content of polyphenolic constituents and antioxidant activity of some *Stachys* taxa. Food Chemistry

104:1277-1281.

Chapter 2 Chickweed

Chandra S and Rawat DS 2015. Medicinal plants of the family Caryophyllaceae: a review of ethno-medicinal uses and pharmacological properties. Integrative Medicine Research 4(3) 123-131.

Chen X-R et al. 2005. Studies on Chemical Constituents of *Stellaria media*. Research and Practice of Chinese Medicines 2005-04.

Chidrawar VR et al. 2011. Anti-obesity effect of *Stellaria media* against drug induced obesity in Swiss albino mice. Pharmacological research 32 (4); 576-584 435.

Hoffmann D 2003. Medical herbalism: the science and practice of herbal medicine. Inner Traditions/Bear and Co, Vermont.

Huang Y et al. 2007. Studies on the Chemical Constituents From *Stellaria Media* (II). Pharmaceutical Journal of the Chinese People's Liberation Army. 2007-03.

Hu Y-M et al. 2005. Aqueous Constituents from *Stellaria Media* (L.) Cyr. Journal of China Pharmaceutical University 2005-06.

Hu Y-M et al. 2009. New triterpenoid from *Stellaria media* (L.) Cyr. Natural Product Research 23, 2009; 14.

Khare CP 2007. Indian Medicinal Plants, An Illustrated Dictionary. Springer-Verlag, Berlin/Heidelberg 219; 508, 583.

Pande A et al. 1995. Lipid constituents from *Stellaria media.* Phytochemistry 39(3) 1995; 709-711.

Shinwari MI and Khan MA. 2000. Folk use of Medicinal herbs of Margalla Hills National Park, Islamabad. J ethnopharmacol 69; 45-56.

Chapter 3 Horsetail

Alexandru V et al. 2007. Investigation of pro-apoptotic activity of *Equisetum arvense* L water extract on human leukaemia U 937 cells. Rouman Biotech Lett 2007; 12(2): 3139-3147.

Canadanovic-Brunet 2008. Radical scavenging and antimicrobial activity of horsetail (*Equisetum arvense* L) extracts. Food Science Technology 44 (2); 269-278.

Carneiro DM et al. 2014. Randomised, double-blind clinical trial to assess the acute diuretic effect of *Equisetum arvense* (Field Horsetail) in healthy volunteers. Evidence-based complementary and alternative medicine vol 2014 Article ID 760683, http://dx.doi.org/10.1155/2014/760683.

Hoffmann Martins do Monte et al. 2004. Anti-nociceptive and anti-inflammatory properties of the hydro-alcoholic extract of stems from *Equisetum arvense* L in mice. Pharmacological Research 49 (3); 239-243.

Hassane M et al. 2004. Platelet anti-aggregant property of some Moroccan medicinal plants. J Ethnopharmacol 2004; 94: 317-322.

Kuriyama K et al. 1998. Anti-acne and anti-dandruff compositions containing lignan glycosides and anti-sebum/antibacterial agents. Jpn Kokai Tokkyo Koho 1998;

Monte FHMD et al. 2005. Cognitive enhancement in aged rats after chronic administration of *Equisetum arvense* L. with demonstrated antioxidant properties *in vitro*. Pharmacol Biochem Behav 2005; 81(3): 593-600.

Nagai T et al. 2005. Antioxidative activities of water extract and ethanol extract from field horsetail (*tsukushi*) *Equisetum arvense* L. Food Chemistry 91 (3); 389-394.

Oh H et al. 2004. Hepatoprotective and free radical scavenging activities of phenolic petrosins and flavonoids isolated from *Equisetum arvenses*. J Ethnopharmacol 95 (2-3); 421-424.

Radulovic N et al. 2006. Composition and antimicrobial activity of *Equisetum arvense* L. essential oil. Phytotherapy research 20 (1); 85-88.

Samura BA and Dovzhenok IA. Influence of plant collections with horsetail field on nervous system. Fiziologichno Aktivni Rechovini 2002; 2: 104-107.

Soleimani S et al. 2007. The effect of *Equisetum arvense* L.

(Equisetaceae) in histological changes of pancreatic β- cells in streptozotocin induced Diabetic in rats. Pak j of biol sci 2007; 10(23): 4236-4240.

Takatsuto S and Abe H 1992. Sterol composition of Strobilus of *Equisetum arvense* L. Biosci Biotech Biochem 1992; 56(5): 834-835.

Yu YB et al. 1998. Screening of some plants for inhibitory effects on HIV-1 and its essential enzymes. Korean J Pharmacog 1998; 29 (4): 338-346.

Zhang G A 2006. Chinese medicinal composition for treating haemorrhoids. Faming Shuanli Shenqing Gonkai Shuomingshu.

Chapter 4 Juniper

Barnes J et al. 2007. Herbal Medicine. 3rd edition. London Pharmaceutical Press.

Carroll JF 2011. Essential oils of *Cupressus funebris, Juniperus communis*, and *J. chinensis* (Cupressaceae) as repellents against ticks (Acari: Ixodidae) and mosquitoes (Diptera: Culicidae) and as toxicants against mosquitoes. Journal of Vector Ecology 36 (2); 258-268.

Foster S et al. 2006. Desk Reference to Nature's Medicine. Washington DC: National Geographic.

German Commission E.

Gordien 2009. Anti-mycobacterial terpenoids from *Juniperus communis* L. (Cuppressaceae) Journal of Ethnopharmacology 126 (3) 2009; 500-505.

Health 2008. Canada Natural Health Products Directorate. Juniper in NHPD Compendium of Monographs. Ottawa, ON; Natural Health Products directorate. April 21 2008.

HerbalGram 2009; 82; 1-2 Juniper Berry, American Botanical Council:

Mabey R 1988. New Age Herbalist, the Fireside.

Miceli N 2009. Comparative Analysis of Flavonoid Profile, Antioxidant and Antimicrobial Activity of the Berries of *Juniperus communis* L. var. *communis* and *Juniperus communis* L. var. *saxatilis* Pall. from Turkey. J. Agric. Food Chem., 2009, 57 (15); 6570–6577.

Nakanishi et al. 2004. Neolignan and flavonoid glycosides in *Juniperus communis* var. *depressa*. <u>Phytochemistry</u> 65(2) 2004; 207-213.

Robbers J E. and Tyler VE 1999. "Tylers Herbs of Choice" Hawthorn Herbal Press.

Shamir F et al 2003. Secretory elements of needles and berries of *Juniperus communis* L. ssp. *communis* and its volatile constituents. Flavour and fragrance journal 18 (5); 425-428.

Chapter 5 Marshmallow

Blaschek W and Franz G 1986. A convenient method for the quantitative determination of mucilage polysaccharides in *Althaea Radix*. Planta Medica 52:S537.

Blumenthal M et al. 1998. The Complete German Commission E Monographs – Therapeutic Guide to Herbal Medicines. Austin, TX; American Botanical Council: Boston: Integrative Medicine Communication: 1998.

Bradley PR (ed) 1992. British Herbal Compendium, vol 1. British Herbal Medicine Association, Bournemouth.

Bradley PR (ed) 2006. British Herbal Compendium, vol 2. British Herbal Medicine Association, Bournemouth.

Brinkmann J et al. 2003. Safety and efficacy of a traditional herbal medicine (Throat Coat) in symptomatic temporary relief of pain in patients with acute pharyngitis: a multi-centre prospective.

Buechi S et al. 2005. Open trial to assess aspect of safety and efficacy of a combined herbal cough syrup with ivy and thyme (abstract). Forsch Komplementarmed Klass Naturheilkd. December 2005: 12(6): 312-313.

Dzido TH et al. 1991. Computer-aided optimisation of high-performance liquid chromatographic analysis of flavonoids from some species of the genus *Althea*. Journal of Chromatography 550: 71-76.

European Pharmacopoeia Commission. Marshmallow Leaf: Marshmallow Root. In: European Pharmacopoeia 5th Edition, Strasbourg, France: European Directorate for Quality of Medicines and Healthcare. 2006: 1974-1975.

Franz G 1989. Polysaccharides in pharmacy: current applications and future concepts. Planta Medica 55: 493-497.

Grieve MA 1931. A Modern Herbal.

Gudej J 1991. Flavonoids, phenolic acids and coumarins from the roots of *Althaea officinalis*. Planta Medica 57: 284-285.

Gudej J. Bieganowska I, 1990. Chromatographc investigations of flavonoid compounds in the leaves and flowers of some species of the genus *Althaea*. Chromatographia 30: 333-336.

Pakravan M et al. 2007. Comparative studies of mucilage cells in different organs in
some species of *Malva* and *Althea*. Pakistan Journal of Biologial Sciences 10: 2603-2605.

Rouhi H and Ganji F 2007. Effect of *Althaea officinalis* on cough associated with ACE inhibitors. Pakistan Journal of Nutrition 6. 256-258.

Seddon B 1965. Submerged peat layers in the Severn Channel near Avonmouth. Proc. Bristol. Nat. Soc. 31.101.

Shimizu N and Tomoda M 1985. Carbon-13 nuclear magnetic resonance spectra of alditol-form oligosaccharides having the fundamental structural units of the Malvaceae plant mucilages and a related polysaccharide. Chemical and Pharmaceutical Bulletin 33: 5539-5542.

Schultz et al. 1998. Rational phytotherapy. Springer-Verlag, Berlin.

Sutovska M et al. 2007. The antitussive activity of polysaccharides from *Althaea officinalis* L, var. Robusta, *Arctium lappa* L var. Herkules, and *Prunus persica* L., Batsch. Bratisl Lek Listy.

2007: 6(3): 256-258.

Wichtl M ed. Brinckmann JA et al 2004. trans Herbal Drugs and Phytopharmaceuticals. Stuttgart: Medpharm Scientific Publishers.

Willems M et al. 2001. How useful is paracetamol absorption as a marker of gastric emptying? A systematic literature study. Digestive Diseases and Sciences. 46: 2256-2262.

Zerehsaz F et al. 2003. Erysipeloid cutaneous leishmaniasis: treatment with a new, topical, pure herbal extract. Eur J Dermatol. March-April 2003: 13(2): 145-148.

Chapter 6 Meadowsweet

Barros L et al. 2011. Chemical, biochemical and electrochemical assays to evaluate phytochemicals and antioxidant activity of wild plants. Food Chemistry 127 (4); 1600-1608.

Boziaris IS et al. 2009. Antimicrobial effect of *Filipendula ulmaria* plant extract against food born pathogenic and spoilage bacteria in laboratory media, fish flesh and fish roe product. Food Technology and Biotechnology 49. 2 (2011): 263.

Calliste C-A 2001. Free Radical Scavenging Activities Measured by Electron Spin Resonance Spectroscopy and B16 Cell Antiproliferative Behaviours of Seven Plants. J. Agric. Food Chem., 2000, 49 (7), pp 3321–3327.

Fluckinger FA 1888. Pharmazeutische Chemie. R. Gaertner's Verlag, Berlin.

Halkes SBA et al. 1997. *In vitro* immunomodulatory activity of *Filipendula ulmaria*. Phytother Res 11 (7) 1997; 518-520

Kahkonen MP et al. 1999. Antioxidant Activity of Plant Extracts Containing Phenolic Compounds. J. Agric. Food Chem., 1999, 47 (10), pp 3954–3962.

Katanic J et al. 2015. Bioactivity, stability and phenolic characterisation of *Filipendula ulmaria* (L.) Maxim. Food Funct., 2015,6, 1164-1175.

Lima MJ 2014. Flower extracts of *Filipendula ulmaria* (L.) Maxim inhibit the proliferation of the NCI-H460 tumour cell line. Industrial Crops and Products 59; 149-153.

Neagu E et al. 2015. Assessment of acetylcholinesterase and tyrosinase inhibitory and antioxidant activity of *Alchemilla vulgaris* and *Filipendula ulmaria* extracts. Journal of the Taiwan Institute of Cheical Engineers 52; 1-6.

Nitta Y et al. 2013. Inhibitory activity of *Filipendula ulmaria* constituents on recombinant human histidine decarboxylase. Food Chemistry 138 (2-3) 2013; 1551-1556.

Papp I et al. 2008. Monitoring Volatile and Non-Volatile Salicylates in *Filipendula ulmaria* by Different Chromatographic Techniques. Chroma (2008) 68: 125.

Rainsford KD 1984. Aspirin and the Salicylates. Butterworth, London, 1984.

Shilova IV 2006. Antioxidant properties of extracts from the above-ground parts of *Filipendula ulmaria*. Pharmaceutical Chemistry Journal 40 (12); 660-662.

Wichtl M and Bisset NG 1994. Herbal Drugs and Phytopharmaceuticals. Medpharm Scientific Publishers, Stuttgart.

Chapter 7 Mugwort

Bahorun T et al. in 2004. Total phenol, flavonoid, proanthocyanidin and vitamin C levels and antioxidant activities of Mauritian vegetables. Journal of the Science of Food and Agriculture 84: 1553-1561.

Blagojevic P et al. 2006. Chemical composition of the essential oils of Serbian wild growing *Artemisia absinthium* and *Artemisia vulgaris*. Journal of Agricultural and Food Chemistry 54: 4780-4789.

Bradley PR 2006. British herbal compendium, vol 2. British Herbal Medicine Association, Bournemouth.

Brooke E 1992. A woman's book of herbs. The Women's Press London.

Wood C Mugwort – Magical Herb of the Moon Goddess.

Fraisse D et al. 2003. Hydroxycinnamic acid levels of various batches from mugwort flowering tops. Annales Pharmaceutiques Francaises 61: 265-268

O Dowd MJ 2001. The history of medications for women. Parthenon Publishing Group, London.

Judzentiene A and Buzelyte J 2006. Chemical composition of essential oils of *Artemisia vulgaris* L (mugwort) from North Lithuania. Chemija 17: 12-15.

Jerkovic I et al. 2003. Chemical variability of *Artemisia vulgaris* L. essential oils originated from the Mediterranean area of France and Croatia. Flavour and Fragrance Journal 18: 436-440.

Kurtzhals JA 2005. Ineffective change of anti-malaria prophylaxis to *Artemisia vulgaris* in a group travelling to West Africa. Ugeskrift for Laege 167: 4082-4083.

Lee SJ et al. 1998. Estrogenic flavonoids from *Artemisia vulgaris* L Journal of Agricultural and Food Chemistry 46: 3325-3329.

Mucciarelli M et al. 1995. Essential oils from some *Artemisia* species growing spontaneously in North-West Italy. Flavour and Fragrance Journal 10: 25-32.

Murray RDH and Stefanovic M 1986. 6-Methoxy-7-8-methylenedioxycoumarin from *Artemisia drancunculoides* and *Artemisia vulgaris*. Journal of Natural Products 49: 550-551.

Nano GM et al. 1976. On the composition of some oils from *Artemisia vulgaris*. Planta Medica 30: 209-215.

Nikolova M 2006. Infraspecific variability in the flavonoid composition of *Artemisia vulgaris* L. Acta Botanica Croatica 65: 13-18.

Weed S. www.susunweed.com

Chapter 8 Great Mullein

Aboutabl EA et al. 1999. Analysis of certain plant polysaccharides and study of their anti-hyperlipidemic activity, Al-Azhar J.

Pharm. Sci. 24, 187-195.

Allen DE and Hatfield G 2004. Medicinal plants in folk tradition,Timber Press, Cambridge, UK.

Ansari S and Daehler CC 2000. Common mullein (*Verbascum thapsus*): A literature review. Pacific cooperative studies unit technical report #127. University of Hawaii at Manoa, Honolulu, USA.

Bom I et al.1998. Hybrid affinity chromatography of α-galactosidase from *Verbascum thapsus* L.J. Chromatogr. A. 808, 133-139.

Bown D 1995. Encyclopaedia of herbs and their uses. Dorling Kindersley, London, U. K.

Carthy ME and Mahony JMO 2010. What's in a name? Can Mullein weed beat TB? Where modern drugs are failing? Evid-Based. Compl. Alt. Doi 10.1155/2011/239237.

Chen RC 2002. Effect of iso-verbascoside, a phenyl-propanoid glycoside antioxidant, on proliferation and differentiation of human gastric cancer cell. www.cnki.com.cn 2002-11.

Coles 1657. Adam in Eden.

Cyr B 2002. Plant extracts and composition containing extracellular protease inhibitors, PCT International Patent WO 02 69,992.

Danchul TY et al. 2007. Flavonoids of some species of the genus *Verbascum* (Scrophulariaceae). Rastitel'nye Resursy. 43, 92-102.

Deng M et al. 2008. Verbascoside rescues the SHSY5Y neuronal cells from MPP-induced apaptosis. Chinese Pharmacological Bulletin 2008-10

Dulger B et al. 2002. Antimicrobial activity of three endemic *Verbascum* species. Pharm. Biol. 40, 587-589.

Grieve M 1981. A Modern Herbal, vol. 2. Dover publications, Inc, New York, pp. 562-566.

Groeger D and Simchen P 1967. Iridoidal plant substances. Pharmazie 22, 315-321.

Halvorson, W.L., Guertin, P., 2003. Fact sheet for: *Verbascum thapsus* L. University of Arizona, Biological Sciences East Tucson, Arizona, USA.

Hattori S and Hatanaka S 1958. Oligosaccharides in *Verbascum thapsus* L. Bot. Mag. Tokyo. 71, 417-424.

Hussain H et al 2009. Minor chemical constituents of *Verbascum thapsus*. Biochem. Syst. Ecol. 37, 124-126.

Ito M et al. 2007. Hair tonics containing natural products. Jpn. Kokai Tokkyo Koho. Patent No. JP2007008885.

Jain SP and Puri HS 1984. Ethnomedicinal plants of Jaunsar-Bawar Hills, Uttar Pradesh, India. J. Ethnopharmacol. 12, 213-222.

Kawamo H et al. 1988. Isolation of an antihistamine flavone from a plant, *Verbascum thapsus*, Jpn. Kokai Tokkyo Koho JP Patent 63,227,584 (88,227,584).

Khan AM et al. 2011. Antimicrobial activity of selected medicinal plants of Margalla Hills, Islamabad, Pakistan. J. Med. Plants Res. 5, 4665-4670.

Kumar GP and Singh SB 2011. Antibacterial and antioxidant activities of ethanol extracts from trans Himalayan medicinal plants. Eur. J. Appl. Sci. 3, 53-57.

Li JX 1999. Effect of verbascoside on decreasing concentration of oxygen free radicals and lipid peroxidation in skeletal muscle. www.cnki.com.cn 199-02

Liao F et al. 1999. Retardation of muscle fatigue by verbascoside and martynoside. Chinese Journal of Pharmacology and Toxicology. 1999-04.

Lin LT et al. 2002. *In vitro* anti-hepatoma activity of fifteen natural medicines from Canada. Phytother. Res. 16, 440-444.

Lyte 1578. The Niewe Herball.

Mahek A et al. 2011. Pharmacognostical standardisation and physico-chemical valuations of leaves of *Verbascum thapsus* Linn. Int. J. Drug Dev. Res. 3, 334-340.

Mccune LM, Johns T 2002. Antioxidant activity in medicinal

plants associated with the symptoms of diabetes mellitus used by the Indigenous Peoples of the North American boreal forest. J. Ethnopharmacol. 82, 197-205.

McCutcheon AR et al. 1995. Antiviral screening of British Columbian medicinal plants. J. Ethnopharmacol. 49, 101-110.

Mehdinezhad B et al. 2011. Comparison of *in-vivo* wound healing activity of *Verbascum thapsus* flower extract with zinc oxide on experimental wound model in rabbits. Adv. Environ. Biol. 5, 1501-1509.

Mehrotra R et al. 1989. Verbacoside. A new luteolin glycoside from *Verbascum thapsus*. J. Nat. Prod. 52, 640-643.

Meurer-Grimes B et al. 1996. Antibacterial activity in medicinal plants of the Scrophulariaceae and Acanthaceae. Int. J. Pharmacogn. 34, 243-248.

Muenscher WC 1935. Weeds. Macmillan Publishing Company, Inc., New York, USA.

Murakami S 1940. Constitution of verbascose, a new pentasaccharide. Proc. Imper. Acad. Tokyo. 16, 12-14.

Murbeck S 1933. Monographie der Gattung *Verbascum*. Acta Univ. Lund ser 2, 29.

Niaz A 2012. Anthelmintic and relaxant activities of *Verbascum Thapsus* Mullein. *BMC* Complementary and Alternative Medicine. The official journal of the International Society for Complementary Medicine Research (ISCMR) 201212: 29

Nichols DG 1887. Medical compound for asthma, etc. (USA). US Patent US00374491.

Obdulio F and Lobete MP 1943. Distribution of rotenone in *Verbascum thapsus*. Farmacia Nueva. 8, 204-206.

Ohara M et al. 2001. Cosmetics, bath preparations, and detergents containing plant extracts. Jpn. Kokai Tokkyo Koho. Patent JP2001122730.

Ota MY et al. 1999. Antioxidants containing *Verbascum* plant extracts and cosmetics containing the extracts. Jpn. Kokai Tokkyo Koho, Patent. JP11171723.

Pande CS and Tewari JD 1960. Chemical examination of the fruits of *Verbascum thapsus*. I. Study on the fat. J. Oil Technol. Assoc. 16, 5-8.

Pardo F et al. 1998. Phytotoxic iridoid glucosides from the roots of *Verbascum thapsus*. J. Chem. Ecol. 24, 645-653.

Parry J et al. 2006. Characterization of cold-pressed onion, parsley, cardamom, mullein, roasted pumpkin, and milk thistle seed oils. J. Am. Oil. Chem. Soc. 83,847-854.

Pascual T et al. 1978a. Components of *Verbascum thapsus* L. I. Triterpenes. An. Quim. 74, 311-314.

Pascual T et al. 1978b. Componentes Del *Verbascum thapsus* L. II. Aceite de las semillas. An. Quim. 78C, 107-110.

Pascual T et al. 1980. Components of *Verbascum thapsus* L. III. Contribution to the study of saponins. An. Quim. Ser. C. 76, 107-110.

Petrichenko VM and Razumovskaya TA 2004. Composition of fatty acids from seeds of three *Verbascum* L. species grown in the Perm region. Rastitel'nye Resursy. 40, 72-77.

Petrichenko VM and Yagontseva TA 2006. Macro and micro elemental composition of genus *Verbascum* (Scrophulariaceae) species in Perm region. Rastitel'nye Resursy. 42, 82-89.

Prior 1870. The Popular Names of British Plants. Williams and Norgate.

Rajbhandari M et al. 2009. Antiviral activity of some plants used in Nepalese traditional medicine. Evid-Based. Compl. Alt. 6, 517-522.

Riaz M et al. 2013. Common mullein, pharmacological and chemical aspects. Rev Bras. Farmacogn. 23 (6) Curitiba nov/ Dec 2013 http://dx.doi.org/10.1590/S0102-6952013000600012

Roia FCJ 1966. The use of plants in hair and scalp preparations. Econ. Bot. 20, 17-30.

Sarrell EM et al. 2001. Efficacy of naturopathic extracts in the management of ear pain associated with acute otitis media. *Archives of Pediatrics and Adolescent Medicine* 2001; 155(7): 796-

9.

Sarrell EM et al. 2003. Naturopathic treatment for ear pain in children. Pediatrics. 111, 574-579.

Seifert K et al 1985. Iridoids from *Verbascum* species. Planta Med. 51, 409-411.

Skwarek T 1979. Effect of some vegetable preparations on propagation of the influenza viruses, II attempts at interferon induction. Acta Pol. Pharm. 36, 715-720.

Souleles C and Geronikaki A 1989. Flavonoids from *Verbascum thapsus*. Sci. Pharm. 57, 59-61.

Speranza L et al. 2010. Anti-inflammatory effects in THP-1 cells treated with verbascoside. Phytother. Res. 24, 1398-1404.

Tatli II and Akdemir ZS 2006. Traditional uses and biological activities of *Verbascum* species. Fabad J. Pharm. Sci. 31, 85-96.

Turker AU and Camper ND 2002. Biological activity of common mullein, a medicinal plant. J. Ethnopharmacol. 82, 117-125.

Turker AU and Camper ND 2002. Biological activity of common mullein, a medicinal plant. Journal of Ethnopharmacology 82 (2-3); 117-125.

Turker AU and Gurel E 2005. Common mullein (*Verbascum thapsus* L.): recent advances in research. Phytother. Res. 19, 733-739.

Verdon E 1912. The pectins of the roots of *Verbascum thapsus* L. and of the leaves of *Kalmia latifolia* L. J. Pharm.Chem. (French). 5, 347-353.

Warashina T et al. 1992. Phenylethanoid and lignan glycosides from *Verbascum thapsus*. Phytochemistry 31, 961-965.

Warashina T et al. 1991. Iridoid glycosides from *Verbascum thapsus* L. Chem. Pharm. Bull. 39, 3261-3264.

Williams JL 1997. Method of treating skin disorders using an extract of mullein. US Patent 08/855, 322.

Yehuda S 2001. PUFA: Mediators for the nervous, endocrine, immune systems, in Mostofsky, DI, Yehuda S, Salem N. (eds). Fatty Acids: Physiological and Behavioural Functions, edited by, Humana Press, Totowa, NJ, pp. 403-420.

Zanon SM et al. 1999. Search for antiviral activity of certain medicinal plants from Cordoba, Argentina. Rev. Latinoam. Microbiol. 41, 59-62.

Zhang C et al. 1996. Studies on the chemical constituents of flannel mullein (*Verbascum thapsus*). Zhongcaoyao. 27, 261-262.

Zhao YL et al. 2011. Isolation of chemical constituents from the aerial parts of *Verbascum thapsus* and their antiangiogenic and antiproliferative activities. Arch. Pharm. Res. 34, 703-707.

Zho HZ 2012. Effects of verbascoside and Martynoside on protecting myocardium and skeletal muscle cell's mitochondria from the damage made by peroxidation in increasing trained rats. Journal of Jinggangshan University (Natural Science) 2012-06.

Zia-Ul-Haq M et al. 2011. Antimicrobial screening of selected flora of Pakistan. Arch. Biol. Sci. 63, 691-695.

Chapter 9 Oak

Alkofahi A and Atta AH 1999. Pharmacological screening of the anti-ulcerogenic effects of some Jordanian medicinal plants in rats. J Ethnopharmacol 67 (3): 341-345.

Andrenšek S et al. 2004. Antimicrobial and anti-oxidative enrichment of oak (*Quercus robur*) bark by rotation planar extraction using Extra Chrom R. Int J Food Microbiol 92(2).181-187.

Carbonaro M et al. 2001. Evaluation of polyphenol bioavailability in rat small intestine. European Journal of Nutrition 40 (2); 84-90.

EMA/HMPC/3206/2009. 25 November 2010. Committee on Herbal Medicinal Products (HMPC). Assessment report on *Quercus robur* L., *Quercus petraea* (Matt.) Liebl., *Quercus pubescens* Willd., cortex. Based on Article 16d (1), Article 16f and Article 16h of Directive 2001/83/EC as amended (traditional use).

Chung KT et al. 1998. Tannins and human health: a review. Crit

Rev Food Sci Nutr 38 (6)421-64.

Fridrich D et al. 2008. Oak ellagitannins suppress the phosphorylation of the epidermal growth factor receptor in human colon carcinoma cells. J. Agric. Food Chem. 56 (9), 3010–3015.

Herve Du Penhoat CL 1991. Structural elucidation of new dimeric ellagitannins from *Quercus robur* J. Chem. Soc., Perkin Trans. 1.

Khennouf S et al. 2003. Effect of tannins from *Quercus ruber* and *Quercus coccifera* leaves on ethanol-induced gastric lesions in mice. J. Agric Food Chem. 51 (5); 1469-1473.

Mohan D et al. 2008. Fungicidal values of bio-oils and their lignin-rich fractions obtained from wood/bark fast pyrolysis. Chemosphere 71 (3); 456-465.

Pallenbach E et al. 1993. Proanthocyanidins from *Quercus petraea* Bark. Planta Med 59(3): 264-268

Piwowarski J P 2014. Role of human gut microbiota metabolism in the anti-inflammatory effect of traditionally used ellagitannin-rich plant materials. J Ethnopharmacol 155; 801-809.

Rivas-Arreola MJ and Rocha-Guzman NE. 2010. Antioxidant activity of oak (*Quercus*) leaves infusions against free radicals and their cardio-protective potential. Pakistan J Biological Sciences. 13 (11); 537-545.

Salminen JP. 2004. Seasonal variation in the content of hydrolysable tannins, flavonoid glycosides and proanthocyanidins in oak leaves. Journal of Chemical Ecology, 30 (9).

Schofield et al. 2001. 25 EMA/HMPC/3206/2009 Committee on Herbal Medicinal Products (HMPC) Assessment report on *Quercus robur* L., *Quercus petraea and Quercus pubescens Willd.*, cortex. Based on Article 16d (1), Article 16f and Article 16h of Directive 2001/83/EC as amended (traditional use).

Uddin G and Rauf A 2012. Phytochemical Screening, Antimicrobial and Antioxidant Activities of Aerial Parts of *Quercus robur* L. Middle-East Journal of Medicinal Plants Research 1(1): 01-04.

Verhaeien EHC and Lemli J 1986. The effect of gallotannins and (+)-catechin on the stimulated fluid secretion on the colon, following a rhein perfusion in guinea pigs. Planta Med (4): 269-72.

Yamasaki H et al. 2007. Antiviral effect of octyl gallate against influenza and other RNA viruses. Int J Molecular Medicine 19: 685-688.

Chapter 10 Raspberry

Anttonen MJ and Karjalainen RO 2005. Environmental and genetic variations of phenolic compounds in red raspberry. Journal of Food Composition and Analysis 18: 759-769.

Bamford DS et al. 1970. Raspberry leaf tea: a new aspect to an old problem British Journal of Pharmacology 40: 205-216.

Beekwilder J et al. 2005a. Antioxidants in raspberry: on-line analysis links antioxidant activity to a diversity of individual metabolites. Journal of Agriculture and Food Chemistry 53: 3313-3320.

Beekwilder J et al. 2005b. Identification and dietary relevance of antioxidants from raspberry. Biofactors 23: 197-205.

Forster DA et al. 2006. Herbal medicine use during pregnancy in a group of Australian women. BMC Pregnancy and childbirth 6:21. Online Available: http://www.biomedcentral.com/bmcpregnancychildbirth/.

Gudej J and Tomczyk M 2004. Determination of flavonoids, tannins and ellagic acid in leaves from Rubus L species. Archives of Pharmacol Research 27: 1114-1119.

Johnson J et al. 2009. Effect of maternal raspberry leaf consumption in rats on pregnancy outcome and the fertility of the female offspring Reproductive Sciences 16: 153-157.

Liu M 2002. Antioxidant and Antiproliferative Activities of Raspberries. J Agric and Food Chem. 50 (10), pp 2926–2930.

Lowdog T 2005. Women's health in complementary and integrative medicine Elsevier. Philadelphia.

Mazu SP 2014. Quality and chemical composition of ten red raspberry (*Rubus idaeus* L.) genotypes during three harvest seasons. Food Chemistry 160; 233-240.

Mc Farlin BL et al. 1999. A national survey of herbal preparation use by nurse midwives for labor stimulation. Review of the literature and recommendations for practice Journal of Nurse-Midwifery 44: 205-216.

Patel AV et al. 2004. Therapeutic constituents and actions of *Rubus species*. Current Medicinal Chemistry 11: 1501-1512.

Puupponen-Pimia R et al. 2005. Berry phenolics selectively inhibit the growth of intestinal pathogens. Journal of Applied Microbiology 98: 991-1000.

Ryan T et al. 2001. Antibacterial activity of raspberry cordial *in vitro*. Research in Veterinary Science 71: 155-159.

Scalbert A et al 2005. Dietary polyphenols and the prevention of disease. Critical Reviews in Food Science and Nutrition 45: 287-306.

Simpson M et al 2001. Raspberry leaf in pregnancy: its safety and efficacy in labor. Journal of Midwifery and Women's Health 46: 51-59.

Wang SY and Lin H-S, 2000. Antioxidant activity in fruits and leaves of blackberry, raspberry, and strawberry varies with cultivar and developmental stage. J. Agric. Food Chem., 48 (2); 140–146.

Chapter 11 Red Clover

Atkinson C et al. 2004. The effects of phytoestrogen isoflavones on bone density in women: a double-blind, randomised placebo-controlled trial. Am J Clin Nutr. 79; 326-333.

Cassady J M 1988. Use of a mammalian cell culture benzo(*a*) pyrene metabolism assay for the detection of potential anti-carcinogens from natural products: Inhibition of metabolism by biochanin A, an isoflavone from *Trifolium pratense* L. Cancer Research 1988.

Clifton Bligh P et al. 2001. The effect of isoflavones extracted from red clover (Rimostil) on lipid and bone metabolism. Menopause. 8(4): 259-265.

Duke J 1997. The green pharmacy: New discoveries in herbal remedies for common diseases and conditions from the world's foremost authority on healing herbs. Rodale.

Griffiths K 1998. 6 Phytoestrogens and diseases of the prostate gland. Bailliere's Clinical Endocrinology and Metabolism 12 (4); 625-647.

Howes JB et al. 2003. Effects of dietary supplementation with isoflavones from red clover on ambulatory blood pressure and endothelial function in postmenopausal type 2 diabetes. Diabetes, Obesity and Metabolism. 5: 325-332.

Huntley AL and Ernst E 2003. A systematic review of herbal medicinal products for the treatment of menopausal symptoms. Menopause 10 (5); 465-476.

Jeri A 2002. The use of isoflavone supplement to relieve hot flushes. The Female Patient 27; 45-50.

Ingram DM 2002. A double-blind randomised controlled trial of isoflavones in the treatment of cyclical mastalgia. The Breast 11 (2); 170-174

Jarred A 2016. Induction of apoptosis in low to moderate-grade human prostate carcinoma by red clover derived dietary isoflavones. Cancer Epidemiology, Biomarkers and Prevention. 11; 1689.

Lin L-Z 2000. LC-ESI-MS Study of the flavonoid glycoside malonates of red clover (*Trifolium pratense.*) J Agric Food Chem 48 (2) 354-365.

Onstad D 1996. Whole food companion White River Junction VA; Chelsea Green Publishing.

Powles T 2004. Isoflavones and women's health. Breast Cancer Research 6; 140.

Teede HJ 2003. Atherosclerosis and lipoproteins. Isoflavones reduce arterial stiffness. A placebo-controlled study in men and postmenopausal women. Vascular Biology 23; 1066-1071.

Tice JA 2003. Phytoestrogen supplements for the treatment of hot flashes: the isoflavone clover extract (ICE) study. A randomised controlled trial. JAMA; 290 (2); 207-214.

Van de Weijer P and Barentsen R 2002. Isoflavones from red clover (Promensil) significantly reduce menopausal hot flush symptoms compared with placebo. Maturitas 42; 187-193.

Widyarini S et al. 2001. Isoflavonoid compounds from red clover (*Trifolium pratense*) protect from inflammation and immune suppression induced by UV radiation. Photochem Photobiol 74: 465-470.

Chapter 12 Dog Rose

Chrubasik C et al. 2008. A systematic review on the *Rosa canina* effect and efficacy profiles. Phytother Res. 2008: 22: 725-733.

Cohen M. 2012. Rosehip: an evidence based herbal medicine for inflammation and arthritis. Australian Family Physician. July 2012; 41 (7); 495-498.

Jalali-Heravi M et al. 2008. Development of a method for analysis of Iranian damask rose oil: Combination of gas chromatography-mass spectrometry with chemometric techniques. Analytica Chimera Acta 623: 11-21.

Jari S et al. 2011. Phytotherapy in medieval Serbian medicine according to the pharmacological manuscripts of the Chilandar Medical Codex (15-16th centuries). Journal of Ethnopharmacol 137(1); 601-19.

Kumar N et al. 2008. Reversed phase-HPLC for rapid determination of polyphenols in flowers of rose species. Journal of Separation Science 31: 262-267.

Phetcharat L et al. 2015. The effectiveness of a standardised rose hip powder, containing seeds and shells of *Rosa canina*, on cell longevity, skin wrinkles, moisture and elasticity. Clinical Interventions in Aging 2015; 10; 1849-1856.

Rein E and Winther K 2001. Cholesterol and C-reactive protein is influenced by rose-hip, a randomised, double-blind, placebo-controlled trial. Proceedings from XIV International Symposium on Drugs Affecting Lipid Metabolism; New York, NY: September 9-12, 2001.

Rein E et al. 2004. A herbal remedy, Hyben Vital (stand. powder of a subspecies of *Rosa canina* fruits), reduces pain and improves general wellbeing in patients with osteoarthritis - a double-blind, placebo-controlled, randomised trial. Phytomedicine. 2004: 11(5): 383-91.

Stevensen C.J 1998. Aromatherapy in dermatology. *Clin. Dermatol.* 16, 689–694.

Tabaei-Aghdaei SR et al. 2007. Morphological and oil content variations amongst Damask rose (*Rosa damascena* Mill) landraces from different regions of Iran. Scientia Horticulturae 113: 44-48.

Tsai TH *et al.* 2010. *In vitro* antimicrobial and anti-inflammatory effects of herbs against *Propionibacterium acnes*. *Food Chem.* 119, 964–968.

Velioglu YS and Mazza G 1991. Characterization of flavonoids in petals of *Rosa damascena* by HPLC and spectral analysis. Journal of Agricultural and Food Chemistry 39: 463-467.

Vinokur Y et al. 2006. Rose petal tea as an antioxidant-rich beverage. Cultivar effects. Journal of Food Science 71: 542-547

Warholm O et al. 2003. The effects of a standardised herbal remedy made from a subtype of *Rosa canina* in patients with osteoarthritis: a double-blind, randomised, placebo-controlled clinical trial. Curr Ther Res Clin Exp. 2003: 64(1): 21-31.

West EW ed. Pahlavi Texts, vol 5. Marvels of Zoroastrianism. In: Muller M, ed. Sacred Books of the East; Oxford University Press 1897.

Willich SN et al. 2010. Rose hip herbal remedy in patients with rheumatoid arthritis - a randomised controlled trial. Phytomed. 2010; 17(2): 87-93.

Winther K et al. 2005. A powder made from seeds and shells

of a rose-hip subspecies (*Rosa canina*) reduces symptoms of knee and hip osteoarthritis: a randomised, double-blind, placebo-controlled clinical trial. Scand J Rheumatol. 2005: 34(4): 302-308.

Winther K et al. 2013 Rose hip powder that contains the natural amount of shells and seeds alleviated pain in osteoarthritis of the dominant hand - a randomized, double-blind, placebo-controlled, cross-over trial. Open Journal of Rheumatology and Autoimmune Diseases. 2013; 3; 172-180.

Chapter 13 Shepherd's Purse

Al-Douri NA and Al-Essa LY 2010. A Survey of Plants Used in Iraqi Traditional Medicine. Jordan Journal of Pharmaceutical Sciences, 3(2), 2010, 100-108.

Al-Snafi A E. 2015. The chemical constituents and Pharmacological effects of *Capsella Bursa-pastoris* - A Review. International Journal of Pharmacology & Toxicology; 5(2), 76-81.

Alizadeh H et al. 2012. The study of antibacterial effect of *Capsella bursa-pastoris* on some of gram positive and gram negative bacteria. J Basic Appl Sci Res, 2(7), 2012, 6940-6945.

Bessette BP 2001. Natural products and gynecology. The Canadian Journal of CME, 2001, 57-72.

Bown D 1995. Encyclopedia of Herbs and their uses. New York; DK Publishing Inc 99, 254.

Choi WJ et al. 2014. Anti-inflammatory and anti-superbacterial properties of sulforaphane from Shepherd's Purse. Korean J Physiol Pharmacol, 18(1), 2014, 33-39.

Duke JA and Ayensu ES 1985. Medicinal Plants of China. Reference publications Inc, USA.

Duke JA 1997. The Green Pharmacy. Rodale Press.

East J 1955. The Effect of certain plant preparations on the fertility of laboratory mammals J Endocrinol, 12(4), 1955, 267-272.

El-Abyad MS et al 1990. Preliminary screening of some Egyptian weeds for antimicrobial activity. Microbios, 62(250), 1990, 47-

57.

Ghoreschi K et al. 2011. Fumarates improve psoriasis and multiple sclerosis by inducing type II dendritic cells. J Exp Med, 208(11), 2011, 2291-2303.

Grieve M 1931. A modern herbal, Shepherd's Purse, *Capsella bursa-pastoris*, http://botanical.com/botanical/mgmh/s/shephe47.html

Grosso C et al. 2011. Chemical composition and biological screening of *Capsella bursa-pastoris*. Brazilian Journal of Pharmacognosy, 21(4), 2011, 635-644.

Guil-Guerrero J et al. 1999. Nutritional composition of wild edible crucifer species. J Food Biochem, 23, 1999, 283-294.

Hasan RN et al. 2013. Antibacterial activity of aqueous and alcoholic extracts of *Capsella bursa pastoris* against selected pathogenic bacteria. American Journal of BioScience, 1(1), 2013, 6-10.

Khare CP 2007. Indian medicinal plants, an illustrated dictionary. Springer Science and Business Media, LLC, 119.

Nieboer C et al. 1989. Systemic therapy with fumaric acid derivates: New possibilities in the treatment of psoriasis. J American Academy Dermatol 20 (4) 1089; 601-608.

Kubínova R et al. 2013. Antioxidant activity of extracts and HPLC analysis of flavonoids from *Capella bursa-pastoris* (L.) Medik.Ceska Slov Farm, 62(4), 2013, 174-176.

Kuroda K and Takagi K 1968. Physiologically Active Substance in *Capsella bursa-pastoris*. Nature, 220, 707-708.

Kuroda K and Akao M 1981. Anti-tumor and anti-intoxication activities of fumaric acid in cultured cells. Gann, 72(5), 1981, 777-782.

Kuroda K et al. 1990. Inhibitory effect of *Capsella bursa-pastoris* extract on growth of Ehrlich solid tumor in mice. Cancer Res, 36(6), 1976, 1900-1903.

Lee KE et al. 2013. Effect of methanol extracts of *Cnidium officinale Makino* and *Capsella bursa-pastoris* on the apoptosis of HSC-

2 human oral cancer cells. Exp Ther Med, 5(3), 2013, 789-792.

Newall CA et al. 1996. Herbal medicines, a guide for herbal care professionals. The Pharmaceutical Press, 1996, 436-437.

Park CJ et al. 2000. Characterization and cDNA cloning of two glycine- and histidine-rich antimicrobial peptides from the roots of shepherd's purse, *Capsella bursa-pastoris*. Plant Mol Biol, 44(2), 2000, 187-197.

Potter's New Cyclopedia of Botanical Drugs and Preparations 1907. Daniel and Co Ltd.

Schultz et al 1998. Rational Phytotherapy. A Physician's Guide to Herbal Medicine. New York; Springer.

Shipochliev T 1981. Uterotonic action of extracts from a group of medicinal plants. Vet Med Nauki, 18(4), 1981, 94-98.

Soleimanpour S et al. 2013. Synergistic antibacterial activity of *Capsella bursa-pastoris* and *Glycyrrhiza glabra* against oral pathogens. Jundishapur J Microbiol, 6 (8), 2013, 7262.

Kweon MH et al. 1996. Structural characterisation of a flavonoid compound scavenging superoxide anion radical isolated from *Capsella bursa pastoris*. J Biochem Mol Biol, 29, 1996, 423-428.

Song N et al. 2007. Several flavonoids from *Capsella bursa-pastoris* (L.) Medic. Asian Journal of Traditional Medicines, 2, 2(5), 218-222.

Yildirim et al. 2012. *In vitro* antibacterial and antitumor activities of some medicinal plant extracts, growing in Turkey. Asian Pacific Journal of Tropical Medicine, 2012, 616-624.

Zennie TM and Ogzewalla D. 1977. Ascorbic acid and vitamin C content of edible wild plants of Ohio and Kentucky. Econ Bot, 31, 76-79.

Chapter 14 Sphagnum Moss

Beith Mary 1995. Healing Threads: Trad. Medicines of the Highlands and Islands. Edinburgh: Polygon.

Darwin T 1996. The Scots. Herbal Edinburgh Mercat Press.

Dickson and Dickson 2000. Plants and People in Ancient Scotland. 79, 226. Stroud: Tempus Pub.

IFCS Irish Folklore Commission, School's survey 736: 22

Johson A 1960. Trans Br Bryol. Soc., 3, 725-8.

Pakarinen and Tolonen 1977. Sphagnum has been used to trap heavy metal pollutants and water born particles and solutes, such as radionuclides, such as Caesium137 (Oikos, 28, 69-73.

St Claire S 1971. Folklore of the Ulster People. Cork. Mercier Press.

Tibbets TE 1968. Peat resources of the world. In: Proc. Third Int. Peat Congress, Quebec 1968

Chapter 15 Tormentil

Bilia AR et al. 1992. A new saponin from *Potentilla tormentilla*. Planta Medica 58: A723.

Bos MA et al. 1996. Procyanidins from tormentil: antioxidant properties towards lipoperoxidation and anti-elastase activity. Biological and Pharmaceutical Bulletin 19:146-148.

Fecka I et al. 2015. Quantification of tannins and related polyphenols in commercial products of tormentil (*Potentilla tormentilla*.) Phytochem Anal. 2015 Sept Oct.

Geiger C et al 1994. Ellagitannins from *Alchemila xanthochlor* and *Potentilla erecta* Planta Medica 60: 384-385.

Haslam E 1996. Natural polyphenols (vegetable tannins) as drugs: Possible modes of action. Journal of Natural Products 59: 205-215.

Kite GC et al. 2007. Chromatographic behaviour of steroidal saponins studied by high-performance liquid chromatography-mass spectrometry. Journal of Chromatography A 1148: 177-183.

Langmead L et al. 2002. Antioxidant effects of herb therapies used by patients with inflammatory bowel disease: an *in vitro* study.

Moss AD and Chefetz AD 2007. Tormentil for active ulcerative colitis. Journal of Clinical Gastroenterology 41: 797-798

Nelson M and Poulter J 2004. Impact of tea drinking on iron status in the UK: a review. Journal of Human Nutrition and Dietetics 17: 43-54.

Palombo EA 2006. Phytochemicals from traditional medicinal plants used in the treatment of diarrhoea: modes of action and effects on intestinal function. Phytotherapy Research 20: 717-724.

Stachurski L et al. 1995. Tormentoside and two of its isomers obtained from the rhizomes of *Potentilla erecta*. Planta Medica 61: 94-95.

Subbotina MD et al. 2003. Effect of oral administration of tormentil root extract (*Potentilla tormentilla*) on rotavirus diarrhoea in children: A randomised, double blind, controlled trial. Pediatric Infectious Disease Journal 22: 706-710.

Thankachan P et al. 2008. Iron absorption in young Indian women: the interaction of iron status with the influence of tea and ascorbic acid. American Journal of Clinical Nutrition 87: 881-886.

Vennat B et al. 1994. Procyanidins from tormentil: fractionation and study of the anti-radical activity towards superoxide anion. Biological and Pharmaceutical Bulletin 17: 1613-1615

Chapter 16 Violet

Amer A and Mehlhorn H 2006. Repellency effect of forty-one essential oils against *Aedes, Anopheles* and *Culex* mosquitoes. Parasitol Res. 2006; 99 (4); 478-490.

Arora DS and Kaur GJ 2007. Antibacterial activity of some Indian medicinal plants. Journal of Natural Medicines. 2007; 61 (3); 313-317.

Bradley PR 2006. British herbal compendium, vol 2. British Herbal Medicine Association, Bournemouth.

De Bairacli Levy J 1973. Common herbs for natural health. Schocken Books. New York.

Drozdova IL and Bubenchikov RA 2005. Composition and anti-inflammatory activity of polysaccharide complexes extracted from sweet violet and low mallow. Pharmaceutical Chemistry Journal 39: 197-200.

Ebrahimzadeh MA et al. 2010. Antioxidant and free radical scavenging activity of *H officinalis* L *var angustifolius, V odorata, B hyrcana* and *C speciosum*. Pak J Pharm Sci 2010; 23 (1); 29-34.

Elhassaneen Y et al. 2013. Effect of Sweet Violet (*Viola odorata* L) Blossoms Powder on Liver and Kidney Functions as well as Serum Lipid Peroxidation of Rats Treated with Carbon Tetrachloride. J American Science. 2013; 9 (5); 88-95.

Feyzabady Z et al. 2014. Efficacy of *Viola odorata* in treatment of chronic insomnia. Iran Red Crescent Med J 16 (12): e17511.

Gerlach SL et al. 2010. Anticancer and chemo-sensitizing abilities of cycloviolacin 02 from *Viola odorata* and psyle cyclotides from *Psychotria leptothyrsa*. Biopolymers 94 (5); 617-25.

Grieve M 1996. A Modern Herbal. Barnes and Noble New York

Hammami I et al. 2011. Biocontrol of *Botrytis cinerea* with essential oil and methanol extract of *Viola odorata* L. flowers. Archives of Applied Science Research, 2011, 3 (5): 44-51.

Ireland DC et al. 2006. A novel suite of cyclotides from *Viola odorata*: sequence variation and the implications for structure, function and stability. Biochemical Journal 2006; 400 (1); 1-12.

Khattak SG et al. 1985. Antipyretic studies on some indigenous Pakistani medicinal plants. J Ethnopharmacol. 1985; 14 (1); 45-51.

Koochek MH et al. 2003. The effectiveness of *Viola odorata* in the prevention and treatment of formalin-induced lung damage in the rat. J of Herbs, Spices and Medicinal Plants 2003; 10 (2); 95-103.

Kumar V et al. 2009. Evaluation of *in vitro* antimicrobial activity and essential oil composition of ethanol extract of *Viola odorata* leaves. World Journal of Pharmacy and Pharmaceutical Sciences. 2015; 4 (5); 1121-1129.

Lamaison JL et al. 1991. Comparative study of *Viola lutea* Huds,

V calcarata L and *V odorata* L. Plantes Medicinales et Phytotherapie 25: 79-88.

Lindholm P et al. 2002. Cyclotides: a novel type of cytotoxic agents. Mol Cancer Ther. 2002; 1 (6); 365-369.

Monadi A et al. 2013. Evaluation of sedative and pre-anesthetic effects of *Viola odorata* Linn. extract compared with diazepam in rats. Bull. Env. Pharmacol Life Sci. 2013; 2 (7); 125-131.

Qasemzadeh et al. 2015. The effect of *Viola odorata* flower syrup on the cough of children with asthma; a double blind, randomized controlled trial. J Evid Based Complementary Altern Med 20 (4); 287-91.

Siddiqi et al. 2012. Studies on the antihypertensive and antidyslipidemic activities of *Viola odorata* leaves extract. Lipids in Health and Disease 11; 6.

Vishala A et al. 2009. Laxative and toxicity studies of *Viola odorata* aerial parts. Pharmacology online. 2009; 1; 739-748

Werkhoff P et al. 1991. Chirospecific analysis in flavour and essential oil chemistry. B, Direct enantiomer resolution of trans-alpha-ionone and trans-alpha-damascone by inclusion gas chromatography. Zeitschrift fur Lebensmittel-Untersuchung und - Forschung 192:111-115.

Zarrabi M et al. 2013. Comparison of the antimicrobial effects of semipurified cyclotides from Iranian *Viola odorata* against some of plant and human pathogenic bacteria. J Appl Microbiol. 2013; 115 (2); 367-375.

Chapter 17 Watercress

Bremness 1994. Herbs. New York; DK Publishing Inc.

Diamond SP et al. 1990. Allergic contact dermatitis to nasturtium. Dermatol Clin 8(1): 7780.

Duke JA 1992. Handbook of Edible Weeds, CRC Press, Boca Raton.

Fekadu Kassie et al. 2002. The effects of garden and water cress juices and their constituents, benzul and phenethyl isothiocyanates, towards benzo (a)pyrene-induced DNA damage: a model study with the single cell gel electophoresis/Hep G2 assay. Chemical-Biological Interactions 142 (3) 285-96.

Freitas E et al. 2013. Antibacterial activity and synergistic effect between watercress extracts, 2-phenylethyl isothiocyanate and antibiotics against 11 isolates of *Escherichia coli* from clinical and animal source. Lett. Appl. Microbiol. 2013 May 18 doi: 10.1111/lam.12105. Shortcut link to this study: http://science.naturalnews.com/pubmed/23682789.html

Goos et al. 2007. On-going investigations on efficacy and safety profile of a herbal drug containing nasturtium herb and horseradish root in acute sinusitis, acute bronchitis and acute urinary tract infection in children in comparison with other antibiotic treatments. Arzneimittelforschung 2007; 57(4): 238-46.

Hecht SS et al. 1995. Effects of watercress consumption on metabolism of a tobacco-specific lung carcinogen in smokers. Cancer epidmiol Biomarkers Prev 4(8): 877884.

Hecht SS 1996. Chemoprevention of lung cancer by isothiocyanates. Adv Exp Med lBiol 40(1): 111.

Mousa-Al-Reza Hadjzadeh et al. 2015. Effects of hydroalcoholic extract of watercress (*Nasturtium officinale*) leaves on serum glucose and lipid levels in diabetic rats. Indian J Physiol Pharmacol 2015. 59 (2) 223-30.

Rose P et al. 2005. β-Phenylethyl and 8-methylsulphinyloctyl isothiocyanates, constituents of watercress, suppress LPS induced production of nitric oxide and prostaglandin E2 in RAW 264.7 macrophages. Nitric oxide 2005; 12 (4); 237-43.

Sadeghi H et al. 2013. *In vivo* anti-inflammatory properties of aerial parts of *Nasturtium officinale*. Pharm Biol. 2014; 52 (2): 169-74.

Schilcher H 1997. Phytotherapy in Paediatrics: Handbook for Physicians and Pharmacists. Stuttgart: Medpharm Scientific Publishers. 5556.

Tevfik-Ozen 2009. Investigation of antioxidant properties of *Nasturtium officinale* (watercress) leaf extracts. Acta Poloniae Pharmaceutica - Drug Research 66 (2); 187-193.

Thomson B and Shaw I, 2002. A comparison of risk and protective factors for colorectal cancer in the diet of new Zealand Maori and non-Maori. Asian Pac. J. Cancer Prev. 2002; 3(4):319-324.

Part III A Few of the Poisonous Plants Used By the Celts

Chapter 2 Periwinkle

Balestreri R et al. 1987. A double-blind placebo controlled evaluation of the safety and efficacy of vinpocetine in the treatment of patients with chronic vascular senile cerebral dysfunction. J Am Geriatr Soc 1987; 35: 425-30.

Blumenthal M ed. the Complete German Commission E Monographs. American Botanical Council in Cooperation with Integrative Medicine Communications. Boston 1998.

Bonoczk P et al. 2002. Vinpocetine increases cerebral blood flow and oxygenation in stroke patients: a near infrared spectroscopy and transcranial Doppler study. Eur J Ultrasound. 2002; 15: 85-91.

Feigin VL et al. 2001. Vinpocetine treatment in acute ischaemic stroke: a pilot single blind randomized clinical trial. Eur J Neurol. 2001; 8: 81-85.

Fischhof PK et al. Therapeutic efficacy of vincamine in dementia. Neuropsychobiology 1996;34: 29-35.

Gabryel B et al. 2002. Piracetam and vinpocetine exert cytoprotective activity and prevent apoptosis of astrocytes *in vitro* in hypoxia and re-oxygenation. Neurotoxicology; 2002; 23: 19-31.

Gulyas B et al. 2001. The effect of a single-dose intravenous vinpocetine on brain metabolism in patients with ischemic stroke (in Hungarian.) Orv Hetil. 2001; 142:443-449.

Hoffmann D 1990. The New Holistic Herbal, 3rd ed. Shaftesbury, Dorset, UK: Element: 223.

Horvath B et al. 2002. *In vitro* antioxidant properties of pentoxifylline, piracetam and vinpocetine. Clin Neuropharmacol. 2002; 25: 37-42.

Kolarov G et al. 2001. Complex effects of cavinton on climacteric symptoms. Akush Ginekol. 2001; 42:37-41.

Neuss N 1980. The spectrum of biological activities of indole alkaloids. In: Phillipson JD, Zenk MH ed. Indole and biogenetically related alkaloids. London Academic Press; 304-305.

Olah VA et al. 1990. An *in vitro* study of the hydroxyl scavenger effect of Cavinton. Acta Paediatr Hung. 1990; 30:309-316.

Pereira C et al. 2003. Neuroprotection strategies: effect of vinpocetine *in vitro* oxidative stress models. Acta Med Port; 2003; 16:401-406.

Proksa B et al. 1988. Relative configuration and cytotoxic activity of vincarubine: a novel bisindole alkaloid from Vinca minor. Planta Medica 1988; 54:214-218.

Reinecke M 1977. Double-blind comparison of vincamine and placebo in patients with presbyacusis. Arzneimittelforschung 1977; 27: 1294-8.

Ribari et al. 1976. Ethyl apovincaminate in the treatment of sensorineural impairment of hearing. Arzneimittelforschung 1976; 26: 1977-80.

Santos M et al. 2000. Synaptosomal response to oxidative stress: effect of vinpocetine. Free Radic Res. 2000; 32: 57-66.

Szilagyi G et al. 2005. Effects of vinpocetine on the redistribution of cerebral blood flow and glucose metabolism in chronic ischemic stroke patients: a PET study. J Neurol Sci. 2005; 229-230: 275-284.

Truss M et al. 2000. Initial clinical experience with the selective phosphodiesterase-I isoenzyme inhibitor vinpocetine in the treatment of urge incontinence and low compliance bladder.

World J Urol. 2000; 18:439-443.

Vas A and Gulyas B 2005. Eburnamine derivatives and the brain. Med Res. Rev. 2005; 25: 737-757.

Chapter 3 Opium poppy

Duke JA 1983. Amerindian Medicinal Plants.

Duke JA 1973. Utilization of Papaver. Econ. Bot. 27(4): 390–391.

Kennedy M 2012. Silchester Iron Age Finds Reveal Secrets of pre-Roman Britain. Guardian 31 July 2012

The Physicians of Myddvai. Translated by John Pughe. 1993 Llanerch.

World Health Organisation 1996. Cancer Pain Relief: with a guide to opioid availability.

Part IV The Roman Invasion

Aldhouse-Green A 2000. Seeing the Wood for the Trees: Symbolism of Trees and Wood in Ancient Gaul and Britain. Aberystwyth: Centres for Advanced Welsh and Celtic Studies. University of Wales, Aberystwyth Research Paper No 17.

Aldhouse-Green A 2006. Boudica Britannia. Pearson, Harlow.

Andouze F and Buchsenschutz O 1992. Towns, Villages and Countryside of Celtic Europe from the Beginning of the Second Millenium to the end of the First Century BC, Translated Henry Cleere BCA.

Caesar J. De Bello Gallico, Commentaries on the Gallic War translated by WA Mc Devitte and WS Bohn 1869. Harper and Brothers New York.

Champlin E 1991. Final Judgements: Deity and Emotion in Roman Wills, 200 BC-AD 250. Berkley: University of California Press.

Cunliffe B 2001. Pytheas the Greek. Penguin.

Graves R 1948. The White Goddess: a Historical Grammar of Poetic Myth. Faber and Faber

Miles D 2005. The Tribes of Britain. Phoenix.

Kennedy M 2012. Silchester Iron Age Finds Reveal Secrets of pre-Roman Britain. Guardian 31July.

Koch JT 2014. Once again Herodotus the Keltoi, the source of the Danube, and the Pillars of Hercules, in Gosden et al. (eds) 2014, 6-18

The Physicians of Myddvai. Translated by John Pughe. 1993 Llanerch

Markale J. Women of the Celts, Translated by A Mygind, C Hauch and P Henry. Gordon Cremonesi 1975.

Matthews C and J 1994. Encyclopaedia of Celtic Wisdom. A Celtic Shaman's Source Book. Element.

Pelletier A 1937. La Femme dans la Société Gallo-Romaine. Paris: Picard.

Pezron P 1703. Antiquite de la Nation, et de la Langue des Celtes, autrement appellez les Gaulois. Paris

Strabo 20 BCE. Geographica.

Zethelius M and Balick M J 1982. Modern medicine and shamanistic ritual: a case of positive synergistic response in the treatment of a snakebite. J Ethnopharmacol 5. 181-185.

Part V

Chapter 1 Celery

Al-Howiriny T et al. 2010. Gastric anti-ulcer, anti-secretory and cytoprotective properties of celery (*Apium graveolens*) in rats. Pharmaceutical Biology 48 (7); 786-793.

Baananou S et al. 2013. Antiulcerogenic and antibacterial activities of *Apium graveolens* essential oil and extract. Nat Prod Res 27 (12); 1075-1083.

Bewick TA et al. 1994. Effects of celery (*Apium graveolens*) root residue on growth of various crops and weeds. Weed Technology 8 (3); 625-629.

Blaszkowski R 2008. US Patent App. 12/244.925.

Butters DE et al. 1999. Extracts of celery seed for the prevention and treatment of pain, inflammation and gastrointestinal irritation. WO oo/40258. 3 November 1999. US Patent 6,352,728, 5 Mar 2002 and Continuation in part as US Patent 6,576,724, 10 June 2003.

Cheng MC et al. 2008. Hypolipidemic and antioxidant activity of Mountain celery essential oil. J Agric Food Chem 2008. 56 (11); 3997-4003.

Deng C et al 2003. Analysis of the volatile constituents of *Apium graveolens* L. and *Oenanthe* L by gas chromatography - mass spectrometry, using headspace solid-phase micro-extraction. Chromatographia 57: 805-809.

Duke J 2003. Green Pharmacy. Rodale.

Friedmen M et al. 2002. Bactericidal activities of plant essential oils and some of their isolated constituents against *Campylobacter jejuni, Escherichia coli, Listeria monocytogenes* and *Salmonella enterica*. J Food Prot 65: 1545-1560

Halim AF et al. 1990 Analysis of celery fruit oil and investigation of the effect of storage. Egyption Journal of Pharmaceutical Sciences 31: 107-113.

Kerishchi P et al. 2011. The effects of *Apium graveolens* extract on sperm parameters and H-G hormonal axis in mice. Proceedings of the International Congress of Physiology and Pharmacology; 2011.

Kittajima J et al. 2003. Polar constituents of celery seed. Phytochemistry 64: 1003-1011.

Ko FN 1991. Vasodilatory action mechanisms of apigenin isolated from *Apium graveolens* in rat thoracic aorta. Biochim Biophys Acta. 1991; 1115 (1); 69-74.

Kooti W and Mansori E 2014. Protective effects of celery (*Apium graveolens*) on testis and cauda epipidymal spermatozoa in rat. Iran J Reprod Med. 2014; 12 (5); 365-366.

Kurobayashi Y et al. 2006. Potent odorants characterise the aroma quality of leaves and stalks in raw and boiled celery. Bioscience, Biotechnology and Biochemistry 70: 958-965.

Lewis DA et al. 1985. The anti-inflammatory activity of celery *Apium graveolens* L (Fam Umbelliferae). Int J Crude Drug Res 23: 27-32.

Lin LZ et al. 2007. Detection and quantification of glycosylated flavonoid malonates in celery, Chinese celery and celery seed by LC-DAD-ESI/MS. Journal of Agricultural and Food Chemistry 55: 1321-1326.

Madkour SO et al. 2014. The beneficial role of celery oil in lowering of di (2-ethylhexyl) phthalate-induced testicular damage. Toxicol Ind Health. 2014. 30 (9); 861-72.

Mencherini et al. 2007. An extract of *Apium graveolens* var. dulce leaves: structure of the major constituent, apiin, and its anti-inflammatory properties. J Pharmacy and Pharmacol 59 (6); 891-897.

Momin RA and Nair MG 2001. Mosquitocidal, nematicidal and antifungal compounds from *Apium graveolens* L seeds. J Agric Food Chem 49: 142-145.

Momin RA and Nair MG 2002. Antioxidant, cyclooxygenase and topoisomerase inhibitory compounds from *Apium graveolens* L seeds. Phytomedicine 9: 312-318.

Pendry B et al. 2005. Phytochemical evaluation of selected antioxidant-containing medicinal plants for use in the preparation of a herbal formula – a preliminary study. Chemistry & Biodiversity 2005; 2 (7): 917-922.

Popovic M et al. 2006. Effect of celery (*Apium graveolens*) extracts on some biochemical parameters of oxidative stress in mice treated with carbon tetrachloride. Phytother Res 20 (7); 531-537.

Shi-Fu M et al. 2007. Hypouricemic action of selected flavonoids in mice: structure activity relationships. Biological and Pharmaceutical Bulletin 30 (8); 1551-1556.

Sturtevant EL 1886. History of celery. The American Naturalist 20: 599-606.

Taher ME et al. 2007. Effects of volatile oil extracts of *Anethum graveolens* and *Apium graveolens* L seeds on activity of liver enzymes in rat. The Journal of Qazvin University of Medical Sciences 11 (2) (43); 8-12.

Vaughan J G and Geissler CA 1997. The new Oxford book of food plants Oxford University Press, Oxford.

Tsi D et al. 2006. Effects of aqueous celery (*Apium graveolens*) extract on lipid parameters of rats fed a high fat diet. Planta Med 1995; 61(1); 18-21.

Tuetun B et al. 2004. Mosquito repellency of the seeds of celery (*Apium graveolens* L). Annals of Tropical Medicine and Parasitology 98 (4); 407-417.

Van Helvoort AL and Van Norren K 2002. US Patent App 20040152640 A1.

Wei A and Shibamoto T 2007. Antioxidant activities and volatile constituents of various essential oils. Journal of Agricultural and Food Chemistry 55:1737-1742.

Whitehouse MW et al. (2000) Anti-inflammatory activity of celery seed extracts in rats with chronic inflammation. Inflammopharmacology 8:310–311

Zidorn C et al. 2005. Polyacetylenes from the apiaceae vegetables carrot, celery, fennel, parsley and parsnip and their cytotoxic activities. J Agric Food Chem 53 (7); 2518-23.

Chapter 2 Elecampane

Bohlmann F et al. 1978. New sesquiterpene lactones from *Inula species*. Phytochemistry 17(7); 1165-1172.

Bree Landwalker: breelandwalker.tumblr.com

British Herbal Medicine Association: British herbal compendium, Bournemouth, 1992, BHMA.

Bourrel C et al. 1993. Chemical analysis, bacteriostatic and fungistatic properties of the essential oil of elecampane (*Inula helenium* L.)Journal of essential oil research 5(4), 411-417.

Cantrell CL et al. 1999. Antimycobacterial eudesmanolides from *Inula helenium* and *Rudbeckia subtomentosa*. Planta Med 65(4):

351-355, 1999.

Encyclopedia of Magical Herbs 1984. Scott Cunningham, Llewellyn

Huo Yan et al. 2012. Chemical constituents of the roots of *Inula helenium*. Chemistry of natural compounds 48(3).

Konishi T et al. 2002. Antiproliferative sesquiterpene lactones from the roots of *Inula helenium*. Biological and Pharmaceutical Bulletin 25 (10); 1370-1372.

Lim SS et al. 2007. Induction of detoxifying enzyme by sesquiterpenes present in *Inula helenium*. J Med Food. 10(3): 503-10.

Luchkova MM 1977. Effect of the anti ulcer drug alantone on gastric mucosa blood circulation in dogs. Fiziolohichnyi Zh 23(5): 1977, 686-687.

Petkova N et al. 2015. Antioxidant activity and fructan content in root extracts from elecampane (*Inula helenium* L.) J. BioSci. Biotechnol. 2015, 4(1): 101-107.

Reiter M and Brandt W 1985. Relaxant effects of *Inula helenium* on tracheal and ileal smooth muscles of the guinea pig. Arzneimittelforschung. 1985; 35(1A):408-14.

O'Shea S et al. 2009. *In vitro* activity of *Inula helenium* against clinical *Staphylococcus aureus* strains including MRSA. Br J Biomed Sci. 2009; 66(4): 186-9

Chapter 3 Garlic

Agarwal KC. 1996. Therapeutic actions of garlic constituents. Med Res Rev. 1996; 16: 111–24.

Amagase H, et al. 2001. Intake of garlic and its bioactive components. J Nutr. 2001; 131: 955–62.

Blumenthal M. The Complete German Commission E Monographs, Special expert committee of the German federal institute for drugs and medical devices, Austin. 1998.

Borek C. Antioxidant health effects of aged garlic extracts. J Nutr. 2001; 131: 1010–5.

Borek C. Garlic reduces dementia and heart-disease risk. J Nutr.

2006; 136: 810–2.

British Pharmacopoeia commission 2007. British Pharmacopoeia London.

Dhawan V and Jain S. Garlic supplementation prevents oxidative DNA damage in essential hypertension. Mol Cell Biochem. 2005; 275: 85–94.

Durak I et al. 2004. Effects of garlic extract consumption on blood lipid and oxidant/antioxidant parameters in humans with high blood cholesterol. J Nutr Biochem. 2004; 15: 373–7.

Durak I et al. 2002. Effects of garlic extract supplementation on blood lipid and antioxidant parameters and atherosclerotic plaque formation process in cholesterol fed rabbits. J Herb Pharmacother. 2002; 2: 19–32.

European Pharmacopoeia 6th Edition 2008. Strasburg: Council of Europe.

Hassan HT 2004. Ajoene (natural garlic compound): a new anti-leukaemia agent for AML therapy. Leuk Res.; 28: 667–71.

Isaacsohn JL et al. 1998. Garlic powder and plasma lipids and lipoproteins: a multicenter, randomized, placebo-controlled trial. Arch Intern Med. 1998; 158: 1189– 94.

Kovacevic N and Beograd Licno Izdanje 2000. Osnovi farmakognozije; pp. 170–1

Ried K et al. 2008. Garlic preparations show benefit in reducing blood pressure. 2008; 8: 13.

Reinhart KM et al. 2008. Effects of garlic on blood pressure in patients with and without systolic hypertension: a meta-analysis. Ann Pharmacother.; 42: 1766–71.

Rohner A et al. 2015. Systematic review and meta-analysis of the antihypertensive effects of garlic. Am J Hypertens. March 2015; 28(3): 414-423.

Sovová M and Sova P 2004. *In vivo* pharmaceutical importance of *Allium sativum* L. 5. Hypolipidemic effects *in vitro* and. Ceska Slov Farm. 2004; 53: 117–23.

Tedeschi P et al. 2007. Fungitoxicity of lyophilized and spray-dried garlic extracts. J Environ Sci Health B. 2007; 42: 795–9.

Ichikawa M et al. 2003. Identification of six phenylpropanoids from garlic skin as major antioxidants. J Agric Food Chem. 2003; 51: 7313–7.

Silagy C and Neil A. Garlic as a lipid lowering agent: a meta-analysis. J R Coll Physicians Lond. 1994; 28: 39–45.

Superko HR and Krauss RM. Garlic powder, effect on plasma lipids, postprandial lipidemia, low-density lipoprotein particle size, high-density lipoprotein subclass distribution and lipoprotein(a) J Am Coll Cardiol. 2000; 35: 321–6.

The United states pharmacopoeial convention. Washington: 2008. USP 31 The United States Pharmacopoeia.

Zhang Y and Yao HP, Huang FF, Wu W, Gao Y, Chen ZB, et al. Allicin, a major component of garlic, inhibits apoptosis in vital organs in rats with trauma/ hemorrhagic shock. Crit Care Med. 2008; 36: 3226–32.

Chapter 4 Lavender

Akhondzadeh L 2003. Comparison of *Lavandula angustifolia* Mill. tincture and imipramine in the treatment of mild to moderate depression: a double-blind, randomized trial. Progress in Neuro-Psychopharmacology and Biological Psychiatry. 27 (1); 123-127.

Basch E et al. 2004. Lavender: Natural Standard Monograph. available at www.naturalstandard.com

Becker RO. The Body Electric. 1985.

Blumenthal M et al. 2000. Herbal Medicine: Expanded Commission E Monographs; Austin TX: American Botanical Council; Newton, MA: Integrative Medicine Communications.

Braun R et al. 2005. eds. Lavendelbluten. In: Standardzulassungen fur Fertigarzneimittel Text and Komentar, mit 16. Erganzungslieferung. Stuttgart, Germany; Deutscher Apotheker Verlag.

Buchbauer G 1991. Aromatherapy: evidence for sedative effects of the essential oil of lavender after inhalation. Zeitschrift fur Naturforschung 46 (11-12); 1067-72.

Cassella S and Smith I. 2002. Synergistic antifungal activity of tea tree (*Melaleuca alternifolia*) and lavender (*Lavandula angustifolia*) essential oils against dermatophyte infection. Int J Aromather 2002; 12 (1); 2-15.

Charron JM 1997. Use of *Lavandula latifolia* as an expectorant (letter) J Altern Complement Med 1997. 3: 211.

D'Auria FD et al. 2005. Antifungal activity of *Lavandula angustifolia* essential oil against *Candida albicans* yeast and mycelial form. Medical Mycology 43, Iss. 5, 2005

DeHart S and Whalen KM 2014. The essential burn book for baristas and cooks; A nurse's fast action secrets to stop pain and miminize blisters. amazon.com Kindle book.

Gattefosse R-M 1910. Aromatherapy.

Ghelardini C et al. 1999. Local Anaesthetic activity of the essential oil of *Lavandula angustifolia*. Planta Med 65 (8); 700-703.

Gismondi A et al. 2014. Biochemical composition and antioxidant properties of *Lavandula angustifolia* Miller essential oil are shielded by propolis against UV radiations. Photochemistry and Photobiology 90 (3); 702-708.

Guillemain J 1989. Neurosedative effects of essential oil of *L angustifolia*. Ann Pharmac Franc 47: 337-343.

Hudson R 1995. Use of lavender in a long term elderly ward. Nursing Times 1995; 91-112.

Hur M and Han SH 2004. Clinical trial of aromatherapy on postpartum mother's perineal healing. Taehan Kanho Hakhoe Chi; February 2004; 34 (1): 53-62.

Jager W 1992. Percutaneous absorption of lavender oil from a massage oil. J Soc Cosmetic Chemists 1992; 43: 49-54.

Kunicka-Styczynska et al. 2015. Preservative activity of lavender hydrosols in moisturizing body gels. Lett Appl Microbiol 60 (1); 27-32.

Lee Y-T 2016. A study of the effect of lavender floral-water eye-mask aromatherapy on the autonomous nervous system. Eur J Integrative Med. 8 (5); 781-788.

Lewith GT et al. 2005. A single-blinded randomized pilot study evaluating the aroma of *Lavandula angustifolia* as a treatment for mild insomnia. J Alternative and Complimentary med. 11 (4); 631-637.

Lis-Balchin M and Hart S 1997. A preliminary study of the effect of essential oils on skeletal and smooth muscle *in vitro*. J Ethnopharmacol 1997; 58: 183-7.

Lis-Balchin M and Hart S 1999. Studies on the mode of action of the essential oil of lavender (*Lavandula angustifolia* P Miller). Phytother Res 1999; 13: 540-2.

Lin PW 2007. Efficacy of aromatherapy (*Lavandula angustifolia*) as an intervention for agitated behaviours in Chinese older persons with dementia: a cross-over randomised trial. Internat J

Geriatric Psychiatry 22 (5); 405-410.

Louis M and Kowalski S 2002. Use of aromatherapy with hospice patients to decrease pain, anxiety and depression and to promote an increased sense of wellbeing. Am J Hosp Palliat Care. Nov-Dec 2002; 19(6): 381-386.

Moon T et al. 2006. Antiparasitic activity of two *Lavandula* essential oils against *Giardia duodenalis, Trichomonas vaginalis* and *Hexamita inflata*. Parasitol Res 99 (6); 722-728.

Morris N 2002. The effects of lavender (*Lavandula angustifolium*) baths on psychological well-being; two exploratory randomised control trials. Complement Ther Med. 2002; 10 (4); 223-228.

Park M and Lee S 2004. The effect of aroma inhalation method on stress responses of nursing students. Taehan Kanho Hakhoe Chi. 2004; 34 (2): 344-351.

Roller S et al. 2009. The antimicrobial activity of high-necrodane and other lavender oils on methicillin-sensitive and resistant *Staphylococcus aureus* (MSSA and MRSA.)

Smith D et al. 2003. Verbal memory elicited by ambient odour. Perceptual and Motor Skills. 2002; 74 (2): 339-343.

Woelk H and Schlafke S 2010. A multi-center, double-blind, randomised study of the Lavender oil prepartion Silexan in comparison to Lorazepam for generalised anxiety disorder. Phytomedicine 2010, 17 (2); 94-99.

Yurkova O 1999. Vegetable aromatic substances influence on oxidative-restoration enzymes state in chronic experiment with animals. Fiziol Zh 199: 45: 40-43.

Zhang Z et al. 1999. Gas chromatographic mass spectrometric analysis of perillyl alcohol and metabolites in plasma. J Chromatogr B Biomed Sci Appl 1999. 728; 85-95.

Zuzarte M et al. 2011. Chemical composition and anti-fungal activity of the essential oils of *Lavandula viridis* L'Her. J Med Microbiol 60: 612-618.

Chapter 5 Marigold

Alexenizor M and Dorn A 2007. Screening of medicinal and ornamental plants for insecticidal and growth regulating activity. J Pestic Sci 2007; 80: 205-215.

Barnes J et al. 2002. Herbal Medicines: A Guide for Healthcare Professionals. London: Pharmaceutical Press; 2002: 103-106.

Bashir S et al. 2006. Studies on spasmogenic and spasmolytic activities of *Calendula officinalis* flowers. Phytother Res 2006; 20; 906-910.

Blumenthal M et al. 2000. Herbal Medicine: Expanded Commission E Monographs; Austin TX: American Botanical Council; Boston: Integrative Medicine Communications.

Bogdanova NS et al. 1970. Study of antiviral properties of *Calendula officinalis*. Farmakol Toksikol (Moscow), 1970; 33; 349.

Chandran PK and Kutton R 2008. Effect of *Calendula officinalis* flower extract on acute phase proteins, antioxidant defence mechanism and granuloma formation during thermal burns. J Clin Biochem Nutr, 2008; 43: 58-64.

Cordova CAS et al. 2002. Protective properties of butanolic extract of *Calendula officinalis* L (marigold) against lipid peroxidation of rat liver microsomes and action as free radical scavenger. Redox Report. Communications in Free Radical Research 7 (2)

Della LR 1990. Topical anti-inflammatory activity of *Calendula officinalis* extracts. Planta Med 1990; 56; 658-658.

Della LR et al. 1994. The role of triterpenoids in topical anti-inflammatory activity of *Calendula officinalis* flowers. Planta Med 1994; 60; 516-520.

Duran V et al. 2005. Results of the clinical examination of an ointment with marigold (*Calendula officinalis*) extract in the treatment of venous leg ulcers. Int J Tissue React 2005; 27 (3):101-106.

Fleisonner AM. Plant extracts; to accelerate healing and reduce inflammation. Cosmet Toilet, 1985; 45; 100-113.

Foster S 2006. National Geographic Desk Reference to Nature's Medicine. Washington DC: National Geographic.

Frankic T et al. 2008. The comparison of *in vivo* anti-genotoxic anti-oxidative capacity of two propylene glycol extracts of *Calendula officinalis* (Marigold) and vitamin E in young growing pigs. J Anim Physiol Anim Nutr, 2008; 41: 1-7.

Fuchs S M et al. 2005. Protective effects of different marigold (*Calendula officinalis* L) rosemary cream preparations against sodium-lauryl-sulfate-induced irritant contact dermatitis. Skin Pharmacol Physiol. July-august 2005: 18 (4):195-200.

Gazim ZC et al. 2008. Antifungal activity of the essential oil from *Calendula officinalis* L (Asteraceae) growing in Brazil. Braz J Microbiol 2008; 39; 61-63.

Goodwin TW 1954. Studies in carotenogenesis; the carotenoids of the flower petals of *Calendula officinalis*. Biochem J, 1954; 58; 90-94

Hoffman D 2003. Medical Herbalism: The Science and Practice of Herbal Medicine. Rochester, VT: Healing Arts Press.

Kalvatene Z et al. 1997. Anti-HIV activity of extracts from *Calendula officinalis* flowers. Biomed and Pharmacother. 1997; 51; 176-180.

Klouchek-Popova E et al. 1982. Influence of the physiological regeneration and epithelialization using fractions isolated from *Calendula officinalis*. Acta Physiologica et Pharmacologica Bulgarica 8(4); 63-67.

Kurkin VA and Sharova OV. 2007. Flavonoids from *Calendula officinalis* flowers. Khim Prir Soed. 2007; 2; 179-180.

Leach MJ 2008. *Calendula officinalis* and wound healing; A systematic review. Wounds 2008; 20 (8); 1-7.

Lievre M et al. 1992. Controlled study of three ointments for the local management of second and third degree burns. Clin Trials Meta-analysis. 1992; 28: 9-12.

Loggia DR et al. 1994. The role of triterpenoids in the topical anti-inflammatory activity of *Calendula officinalis* flowers. Planta Med. 1994: 60: 516-520.

Medina EJ et al. 2006. A new extract of the plant *Calendula officinalis* produces a dual *in vitro* effect: cytotoxic anti-tumor activity and lymphocyte activation. BMC Cancer, 2006: 6: 119-132.

Muley BP et al. 2009. Phytochemical constituents and pharmacological activities of *Calendula officinalis* Linn (Asteraceae): A Review. Tropical Journal of Pharmaceutical Research 2009: 8 (5): 455-465.

Patrick KFM et al. 1996. Induction of vascularisation by an aqueous extract of the flowers of *Calendula officinalis* L the European marigold. Phytomedicine 3 (1); 11-18.

Popovic M et al. 1999. Combined effects of plant extracts and xenobiotics on liposomal lipid peroxidation. Part I. Marigold extract-ciprofloxacin/pyralene. Oxidation Commum. 1999; 22: 487-494.

Preethi K et al. 2008. Effect of *Calendula officinalis* flower extract on acute phase proteins, antioxidant defense mechanism and granuloma formation during thermal burns. J Clin Biochem and Nutrition. 43 (2); 58-64.

Tyler V E 1994. Herbs of Choice: The Therapeutic use of Phyto-medicinals. New York: Pharmaceutical Products Press; 1994.

Ukiya M et al. 2006. Anti-inflammatory and anti-tumour pro-moting and cytotoxic activities of constituents of Marigold (*Calendula officinalis*) flowers. J Nat Prod 2006; 69; 1692-1696.

Varlijen J 1989. Structural analysis of rhamnoarabinogalactans and arabinogalactans with immuno-stimulating activity from *Calendula officinalis*. Phytochemistry, 1989; 28: 2379-2383.

Wichtl M ed 2004. Herbal Drugs and Phytopharmaceuticals. 3rd ed. Stuttgart: Medpharm GmbH Scientific Publishers.

Zitteri-Eglseer K et al. 1997. Anti-oedematous activities of the main triterpendiolesters of marigold (*Calendula officinalis* L.) J Ethnopharmacol 1997; 57 (2); 139-144.

Chapter 6 Rosemary

Abu-Al-Basal M 2010. Healing potential of *Rosmarinus officinalis* L on full-thickness excision cutaneous wounds in alloxan-in-duced-diabetic BALB/c mice. J Ethnopharmacol 131 (2); 443-450.

Atsumi T 2007. Smelling lavender and rosemary increases free radical scavenging activity and decreases cortisol level in sa-liva. Psychiatry Research 150 (2007) 89-96.

al-Sereiti M R and Said S A, 1992. First Medical Conference of Libya.

al-Sereiti MR et al. 1999. Pharmacology of rosemary (*Rosmarinus officinalis* Linn.) and its therapeutic potentials. Indian J Exp Biol. 1999; 37(2); 124-30.

Aqel M B 1991. Relaxant effect of the volatile oil of *Romarinus officinalis* on tracheal smooth muscle. J Ethnopharmacol, 33 (1991) 57.

Bozin B et al. Antimicrobial and antioxidant properties of rose-mary and sage (*Rosmarinus officinalis* L. and *Salvia officinalis*

L., Lamiaceae) essential oils. Journal of Agricultural and Food Chemistry 55.19 (2007): 7879-7885.

Duke JA and Ayensu E S 1985. Medicinal Plants of China.

Durakovic Z and Durakovic S 1979. The effect of rosemary oil on *Candida albicans*. J Indian Med Assoc, 72 (1979) 175.

European Medicines Agency. Committee on Herbal Medicinal Products (HMPC) EMA/HMPC/13631/2009.

Hayashi T et al. 1987. Studies on medicinal-plants in Paraguay – Studies on Romero 1. Planta Med, 52 (1987) 394.

Hoefler C et al. 1987. Comparative choleretic and hepatoprotective properties of young sprouts and total plant extracts of *Rosmarinus officinalis* in rats. J Ethnopharmacol, 19 (1987) 133.

Houlihan C et al. 1985. The structure of rosmariquinone — A new antioxidant isolated from *Rosmarinus officinalis* L.J Am Oil Chem Soc, 62(1985) 96.

Huang MT et al. 1994. Inhibition of skin tumorigenesis by rosemary and its constituents carnosol and ursolic acid. Cancer Res 1994; 54; 701-708.

Johnson J 2011. Carnosol; A promising anti-cancer and anti-inflammatory agent. Cancer Letters 2011. 305 (1); 1-7.

Kimura Y et al. 1987. Studies on the activities of tannins and related compounds, X. Effects of caffeetannins and related compounds on arachidonate metabolism in human. J Nat Prod, 50; 392.

Kosaka K and Yokor T 2003. Carnosic acid, a component of rosemary (*Rosmarinus officinalis* L) promotes synthesis of nerve growth factor in T98G human glioblastoma cells. Biological and Parmaceutical Bulletin 26 (2003) 11P 1620-1622.

Kotb D F 1985. Medicinal plants in Libya (Arab Encyclopedia House, Tripoli); 720.

Kovar K A et al. 1987. Blood Levels of 1, 8-Cineole and Locomotor Activity of Mice After Inhalation and Oral Administration of Rosemary Oil. Planta Med, 53 (1987) 315.

Lo AH et al. 2002. Carnosol, an antioxidant in rosemary, suppresses inducible citric oxide synthase through down-regulating nuclear factor-kappaB in mouse macrophages. Carcinogenesis 2002; 23; 983-991.

Machado DG et al. 2009. Antidepressant-like effect of the extract of *Rosmarinus officinalis* in mice; Involvement of the monoaminergic system. Progress in Neuro-Psychopharmacology and Biological Psychiatry 33 (4); 642-650.

Mahady GB et al. 2005. *In vitro* susceptibility of *Helicobacter pylori* to botanical extracts used traditionally for the treatment of gastrointestinal disorders. Phytotherapy Res 19 (11); 988-991.

Oluwatuyi M et al. 2004. Antibacterial and resistance modifying activity of *Rosmarinus officinalis*. Phytochemistry 65 (24); 3249-3254.

Orhan I et al. 2008. Inhibitory effect of Turkish *Rosmarinus officinalis* L on acetylcholinesterase and butyrylcholinesterase enzymes. Food chemistry 108 (2); 663-668.

Pengelly A et al. 2012. Short-term study on the effects of rosemary on cognitive function in an elderly population. J Medicinal Food. 15 (1) 10-17.

Pintore G et al. 2002. Chemical composition and antimicrobial activity of *Rosmarinus officinalis* L. oils from Sardinia and Corsica. Flavour and Fragrance Journal 2002; 17(1);15-19.

Rasooli I et al. 2008. Antimycotoxigenic characteristics of *Rosmarinus officinalis* and

Trachyspermum copticum L. essential oils. International Journal of Food Microbiology Vol 122; 1-2, 29 Feb 2008; 135-139

Rulffs W 1984. Rosemary oil bath additive. Proof of effectiveness. Munch Med Wochensch, 1984 Feb 24; 126 (8); 207-8.

Santoyo S et al. 2005. Chemical composition and antimicrobial activity of *Rosmarinus officinalis* L. essential oil obtained via supercritical fluid extraction. J Food Protection 4. 2005; 660-884.

Schwarz K et al. 2001. Investigation of plant extracts for the protection of processed foods against lipid oxidation. Comparison of antioxidant assays based on radical scavenging, lipid oxidation and analysis of the principal antioxidant compounds. Eur Food Res Technol 2001; 212; 319-328.

Singletary K W and Nelshoppen J M 1991. Inhibition of 7, 12-dimethylbenz [a] anthracene (DMBA)-induced mammary tumorigenesis and of *in vivo* formation of mammary DMBA-DNA adducts by rosemary. Cancer Lett, 60 (1991) 169.

Solhi H et al. 2013. Beneficial Effects of *Rosmarinus Officinalis* for treatment of opium withdrawal syndrome during addiction treatment programs: A clinical trial. Addiction & Health 2013; 5 (3-4): 90-4.

Soyal D et al. 2007. Modulation of radiation-induced biochemical alterations in mice by rosemary (*Rosemarinus officinalis*) extract. Phytomedicine 14.10: 701-705.

Suong N et al. 2011. Rosemary and cancer prevention: pre-clinical perspectives. Critical Reviews in Food Science and Nutrition 51 (10); 946-954.

Tyler VE 1994. Herbs of Choice: The Therapeutic Use of Phytomedicinals. New York, NY Pharmaceutical Product Press.

Wu J W et al. 1982. Elucidation of the chemical structures of natural antioxidants isolated from rosemary. J Am Oil Chem Soc, 59 (1982) 339.

Yesil Celiktas O et al. 2007. Antimicrobial activities of methanol extracts and essential oils of *Rosmarinus officinalis*, depending on location and seasonal variations Food Chemistry 2007; 100 (2); 553–559.

Chapter 7 Sage

Akhondzadeh S et al. 2003. *Salvia officinalis* extract in the treatment of patients with mild to moderate Alzheimer's disease; a double blind randomised placebo-controlled trial. J Clin Pharm Ther. 2003; 28: 53-59.

Baricevic D et al. 2001. Topical anti-inflammatory activity of *Salvia officinalis* L leaves: the relevance of ursolic acid. J Ethnopharmacol 75 (2); 125-132.

Behradmanesh S et al. 2013. Effect of *Salvia officinalis* on diabetic patients. Journal of Renal Injury Prevention 2013. 2(2); 51-54.

De Leo et al. 1998. Treatment of neurovegetative menopausal symptoms with a phytotherapeutic agent. Minerva Ginecologica 1998; 50(5); 207-211.

Haughton PJ 2004. Activity and constituents of sage relevant to the potential treatment of symptoms of Alzheimer's disease. Herbal Gram 2004; 61: 38-53.

Hauouni EA et al. 2008. Tunisian *Salvia officinalis* L and *Schinus molle* L. essential oils: their chemical compositions and their preservative effects against *Salmonella* inoculated in minced beef meat. Int. J Food Microbiol 125 (3): 242-251.

Kennedy DO et al. 2006. Effects of cholinesterase inhibiting sage (*Salvia officinalis*) on mood, anxiety and performance on a psychological stressor battery. Neuro-psycho-pharmacology. 2006; 31: 845-852.

Kianbakht S et al. 2011. Antihyperlipidemic effects of *Salvia officinalis* L leaf extract in patients with hyperlipidemia: a randomised double-blind placebo-controlled clinical trial.

Kianbakht S et al. 2013. Improved glycemic control and lipid profile in hyperlipidemic type 2 diabetic patients consuming *Salvia officinalis* L leaf extract: a randomised placebo controlled clinical trial. Complementary Therapies in Medicine 21 (5): 441-446.

Longaray Delamare AP et al. 2007. Antibacterial activity of the essential oils of *Salvia officinalis* L and *Salvia triloba* L cultivated in South Brazil. Food Chemistry 2007. 100 (2); 603-608.

Lu Y and Foo LY 2002. Polyphenolics of *Salvia*—a review. Phytochemistry 59; (2002) 117–140.

Moss L et al 2010. Differential effects of the aromas of *Salvia* species on memory and mood. Hum Phychopharmacol. 2010; 25 (5); 388-396.

Pinto E et al. 2007. *In vitro* susceptibility of some species of yeasts and filamentous fungi to essential oils of *Salvia officinalis*. Industrial crops and Products. 2007. 26 (2); 135-141.

Rahte S et al. 2013. *Salvia officinalis* for hot flushes: towards determination of mechanism of activity and active principles. Planta Med 2013. 79 (9); 753-60.

Reuter J et al. 2007. Sage extract rich in phenolic diterpenes inhibits ultra violet induced erythema *in vivo*. Planta Med. 2007; 73(11): 1190-1191.

Saller R et al. 2001. Combined herbal preparation for topical treatment of *Herpes labialis*. Forschende Komplementarmedizin und Klassische Naturheilkunde. 2001; 8; 373-382.

Schapowal A et al. 2009. Echinacea/sage or chlorhexidine/lidocaine for treating acute sore throats: a randomized double blind trial. Eur J Med Res. 2009; 14 (9): 406-412.

Scholey AB et al. 2008. An extract of *Salvia* (sage) with anti-cholinesterase properties improves memory and attention in healthy older volunteers. Psychopharmacology. 2008; 198: 127-139.

Conclusion References

Bell SJ and Sears B 2003. Low-glycemic-load diets: impact on obesity and chronic diseases. Critical Reviews in Food Science and Nutrition, 43 (4); 357-377.

Bowman SA 1999. Diets of individuals based on energy intakes from added sugars. Family Economics and Nutrition Review 12 (2); 31-38

Dental Caries and Its Complications: Tooth Decay. The Marck Manual of Diagnosis and Therapy, edited by Robert Berkow et al. Rahway NJ: Merck Research Laboratories, 1992.

Geerts SO et al. 2004. Further evidence of the association between periodontal conditions and coronary artery disease. Journal of Periodontology, 75 (9) 2004; 1274-80.

Sensi M et al. 1991. Advanced Nonenzymatic glycation endproducts (AGE): Their relevance to aging and the pathogenesis of late diabetic complications. Diabetes Research 16(1); 1-9.

Shock, NW et al 1984. Normal Human Ageing: the Baltimore Longitudinal Study of Ageing. (DHHS/NIH), Bethesda MD.

Weiss EP and Fontana L. 2011. Caloric restriction: powerful protection for the ageing heart and vasculature. Am J Physiol Heart Circ Physiol. 301(4): H1205-H1219

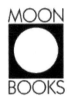

MOON

BOOKS

Moon Books

PAGANISM & SHAMANISM

What is Paganism? A religion, a spirituality, an alternative belief system, nature worship? You can find support for all these definitions (and many more) in dictionaries, encyclopaedias, and text books of religion, but subscribe to any one and the truth will evade you. Above all Paganism is a creative pursuit, an encounter with reality, an exploration of meaning and an expression of the soul. Druids, Heathens, Wiccans and others, all contribute their insights and literary riches to the Pagan tradition. Moon Books invites you to begin or to deepen your own encounter, right here, right now.
If you have enjoyed this book, why not tell other readers by posting a review on your preferred book site. Recent bestsellers from Moon Books are:

Journey to the Dark Goddess
How to Return to Your Soul
Jane Meredith
Discover the powerful secrets of the Dark Goddess and transform your depression, grief and pain into healing and integration.
Paperback: 978-1-84694-677-6 ebook: 978-1-78099-223-5

Shamanic Reiki
Expanded Ways of Working with Universal Life Force Energy
Llyn Roberts, Robert Levy
Shamanism and Reiki are each powerful ways of healing; together,
their power multiplies. Shamanic Reiki introduces techniques to
help healers and Reiki practitioners tap ancient healing wisdom.
Paperback: 978-1-84694-037-8 ebook: 978-1-84694-650-9

Pagan Portals – The Awen Alone
Walking the Path of the Solitary Druid
Joanna van der Hoeven
An introductory guide for the solitary Druid, The Awen Alone
will accompany you as you explore, and seek out your own place
within the natural world.
Paperback: 978-1-78279-547-6 ebook: 978-1-78279-546-9

A Kitchen Witch's World of Magical Herbs & Plants
Rachel Patterson
A journey into the magical world of herbs and plants, filled with
magical uses, folklore, history and practical magic. By popular
writer, blogger and kitchen witch, Tansy Firedragon.
Paperback: 978-1-78279-621-3 ebook: 978-1-78279-620-6

Medicine for the Soul
The Complete Book of Shamanic Healing
Ross Heaven
All you will ever need to know about shamanic healing and how to
become your own shaman...
Paperback: 978-1-78099-419-2 ebook: 978-1-78099-420-8

Traditional Witchcraft for the Woods and Forests
A Witch's Guide to the Woodland with Guided Meditations and
Pathworking
Melusine Draco
A Witch's guide to walking alone in the woods, with guided
meditations and pathworking.
Paperback: 978-1-84694-803-9 ebook: 978-1-84694-804-6

Wild Earth, Wild Soul
A Manual for an Ecstatic Culture
Bill Pfeiffer
Imagine a nature-based culture so alive and so connected,
spreading like wildfire. This book is the first flame...
Paperback: 978-1-78099-187-0 ebook: 978-1-78099-188-7

Naming the Goddess
Trevor Greenfield
Naming the Goddess is written by over eighty adherents and
scholars of Goddess and Goddess Spirituality.
Paperback: 978-1-78279-476-9 ebook: 978-1-78279-475-2

Readers of ebooks can buy or view any of these bestsellers by
clicking on the live link in the title. Most titles are published in
paperback and as an ebook. Paperbacks are available in traditional
bookshops. Both print and ebook formats are available online.

Find more titles and sign up to our readers' newsletter at
http://www.johnhuntpublishing.com/paganism
Follow us on Facebook at https://www.facebook.com/MoonBooks
and Twitter at https://twitter.com/MoonBooksJHP